Praise for *Clean Protein*

"This is the right book at the right time for a nation obsessed with protein . . . Their conversational tone whisks the reader through compelling science to a clear prescriptive toward a healthier you and a better world—through clean protein."

> —Dan Buettner, National Geographic Fellow and *New York Times* Bestselling author of the Blue Zones books

"In an accessible and friendly manner, Kathy and Bruce provide a step-by-step guide to a healthier and happier you. I enjoyed reading this no-nonsense guilt-free guide to where and how we should all be getting our protein, and you will too."

> —Dr. Dean Ornish, president and founder of the nonprofit Preventive Medicine Research Institute and bestselling author of *Dr. Dean Ornish's Program for Reversing Heart Disease, Eat More, Weigh Less* and *The Spectrum*

"My favorite part about this book is its realism; Kathy and Bruce invite everyone into their clean protein vision, starting with Big Food, who Kathy and Bruce see as key partners in a necessary global dietary shift.

> —Michael Greger, founder of NutritionFacts.org and author of the *New York Times* bestseller *How Not to Die: Discover the Foods Scientifically Proven to Prevent and Reverse Disease*

"Read this book! Clean protein is an idea whose time has come . . . Their advice is both great for your health and great for the world!"

> —John Mackey, founder and CEO of Whole Foods and author of *Conscious Capitalism: Liberating the Heroic Spirit of Business*

"Confusion about protein is a crazy issue. We overeat, waste too much and still can't conquer hunger. Freston and Friedrich tell us exactly what kind of protein to eat and how to make it taste delicious."

"[A] powerful and compelling book that will help to catalyze the type of food revolution that is so desperately needed at this point in our world's history. The book is very useful on a personal level, clearly and concisely providing . . . all of the ingredients to allow individuals to easily incorporate clean protein concepts into their daily lives."

"*Clean Protein* cuts through myth and misconception alike . . . This book could scarcely be more needed, important, and timely."

Clean Protein

Also by Kathy Freston:

Quantum Wellness:
A Practical Guide to Health and Happiness

Veganist: Lose Weight,
Get Healthy, Change the World

The Lean: A Revolutionary (and Simple!) 30-Day
Plan for Healthy, Lasting Weight Loss

Clean Protein

The Revolution that will
Reshape Your Body, Boost Your
Energy—and Save Our Planet

Kathy Freston and Bruce Friedrich

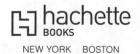

NEW YORK   BOSTON

Hachette Books
Hachette Book Group
1290 Avenue of the Americas, New York, NY 10104
hachettebooks.com
twitter.com/hachettebooks

First Edition: January 2018

Hachette Books is a division of Hachette Book Group, Inc. The Hachette Books name and logo are trademarks of Hachette Book Group, Inc.

The publisher is not responsible for websites (or their content) that are not owned by the publisher.

The Hachette Speakers Bureau provides a wide range of authors for speaking events. To find out more, go to www.hachettespeakersbureau.com or call (866) 376-6591.

Print book interior design by Trish Wilkinson.

Library of Congress Cataloging-in-Publication Data has been applied for.

ISBNs: 978-1-60286-332-3 (hardcover), 978-1-60286-333-0 (e-book)

Printed in the United States of America

LSC-C

10 9 8 7 6 5 4 3 2 1

For Alka and for Dan

Contents

Contents

Introduction

Mark stares into the mirror at a body he hardly recognizes. His muscles appear flaccid, his hair patchy, his skin sagging. He looks and feels exhausted. After a quick Google search, one word surfaces as the answer to his problems: protein. Mark rushes to the store and joins the plethora of Americans in a crusade to eat as much protein as possible. His meal plan for the next day includes two eggs, beans, and bacon for breakfast; a broiled chicken breast with buttered broccoli for lunch; and a hearty hamburger (no bun) with a side of quinoa for dinner. He washes each meal down with a whey-protein shake.

By the time Mark goes to sleep with dreams of his future Adonis-like physique, he's consumed 190 grams of protein—nearly three times the amount suggested by the Institute of Medicine. He's also spent three times more on groceries, from the free-range chicken breasts to the omega-3-fortified eggs to the locally sourced burger meat. But at Mark's next checkup, his doctor informs him that his cholesterol levels have skyrocketed and his blood pressure is off the charts. He is a ticking time bomb, his doctor warns. *Is this what all that protein has given me?* Mark now wonders. *There has to be a better way.*

Diet fads come and go, but they all find their way to Samantha. She has called herself a "professional dieter" ever since her quest for a weight-loss magic bullet became an obsession. Samantha has jettisoned starches from her fridge, which is now overflowing with meat, eggs, and full-fat dairy products. Her favorite is Greek yogurt. Samantha is pleased that so many of her favorite foods, like bacon and heavy cream, are included in the diet she's currently following, all in the name of protein. She isn't sure how much protein she's consuming, but as long as her food comes from something that "swam, flew, or walked," she assumes she's doing the right thing. She lost a dozen pounds on her new diet . . . but then the weight piled back on relentlessly. Meanwhile, she's been so constipated that she needs a daily laxative.

Sally spends most of her time worrying about her five-year-old daughter's well-being. Is she making friends? Is she being challenged in school? Is she . . . getting enough protein? Sally sees constant protein reminders throughout her day. The National Fluid Milk Association runs an ad campaign titled "Milk Life," emphasizing the health benefits of protein consumption (through milk, of course). The National Dairy Council provides classroom materials for her daughter's preschool. Sally knows that protein is a vital part of a child's diet, but she didn't know it was *this* vital. Just the other day, Sally took a picture of her daughter's lunch—a banana, carrots, and her favorite spaghetti with garlic bread—and posted it on Facebook. Sally couldn't believe the comments: "Yum! But where's the protein?!" and "A growing girl needs protein!!!" She feels like a bad mom, and there's no worse feeling than that. She is afraid to ask that simple question: "What's the big deal with protein?" There are collages of people we have heard from throughout the years, but their concern is the same: protein.

Today it seems everyone has an answer for that question, but rarely the right one. The only constant is that we're obsessed with protein. We look for it on menus and labels, form the family table around it, and get anxious at the thought of not eating enough of it. This is for a good reason: protein is essential. It makes your hair strong and your skin supple. It fuels your immune system. It helps form the hormones, neurotransmitters, and enzymes that affect the functioning of your organs and nerves. Protein is, quite literally, the foundational building block of a healthy body. Without it, life would not be possible.

Protein was first isolated in 1839 by a Dutch chemist named Gerhard Mulder. He named his discovery after the Greek word *proteios,* which means "of primary importance." It was a fitting baptism for a nutrient that has become the subject of a nationwide fixation. We need to eat protein to survive, but our supersized culture has twisted this fact into a dangerous fallacy: that we need to eat as much protein as possible.

Mulder originally isolated protein from meat, which gave birth to another myth: that only animal products have protein. That's not the case—there are many sources of protein—but most people are under that impression, perhaps because it's ubiquitous and easy.

Of course animal protein may have been essential long ago for nourishing our ancestors in times of scarcity. These apish humans scavenged for animal meat when there wasn't enough plant food to sustain them, and the extra calories helped hasten human evolution. (Until the invention of tools, early humans were not effective hunters. They had to rely on larger and faster animals to leave fallen prey for them to scavenge.) And even still, a little bit of meat is fine for humans. But you know how we humans tend to be: if a little bit is fine, more must be better.

Speaking about more. . . .

The so-called Green Revolution, which drastically increased the productivity of global agriculture by introducing new chemical fertilizers and synthetic herbicides, is credited with saving more than a billion people from starvation during the mid-twentieth century. The increased yield made it possible to feed a growing human population. This was the intention, anyway, and it was a worthy one. However, although these high-yield crops promised to be a panacea for global hunger, there was at least one additional effect: cheaper and more readily available grains could also make it possible to raise more animals, which meant cheaper meat, dairy, and eggs. Animal products, once a luxury, were now a staple. A profitable staple. Small-scale animal producers continued to raise animals in a traditional, sustainable manner, but they were soon to be trounced by industrial factory farms—corporations—taking advantage of the inexpensive corn, soy, and wheat to mass-produce animals for slaughter.

We soon learned the consequences of cheap, plentiful food with Frances Moore Lappé's groundbreaking 1971 book, *Diet for a Small Planet*. All of that mass production is placing immense pressure on our land, water, and air—not to mention on animals themselves. The inefficiencies of cycling crops through animals are catching up with us, and, as the global population grows and continues to demand more and more protein, we will pass the breaking point. The Food and Agriculture Organization of the United Nations concludes that we're going to have to increase food production by 70 percent if we want to feed the world's population in 2050, which is impossible given our current reliance on land-, water-, and energy-intensive animal agriculture. Quite simply, if we keep producing food like we do now, we will not be able to feed the world's population by midcentury.

We are also reaching a breaking point with our health. A little bit of meat may not be especially harmful, but we are eating far more animal protein than our bodies are capable of handling. As a result, we are plagued by heart disease, cancer, and obesity-related illnesses—all, which you'll see in the upcoming chapters, are closely tied to meat, dairy, and egg consumption. We are a meat culture—or, rather, a *meat protein* culture—and we are only beginning to comprehend the health consequences.

Meanwhile, we've been exporting our animal protein obsession to other countries. In the past four decades, the revved-up, consumer-driven, hungry world has seen demand for meat triple and egg consumption increase sevenfold, causing a vast expansion of degenerative disease—often called "diseases of affluence." Since World War II, egg consumption in Japan has increased sevenfold, meat consumption ninefold, and dairy consumption twentyfold. This correlates with a twenty-five-fold increase in prostate cancer incidences among Japanese men, while rates of Alzheimer's disease among men and women have increased sevenfold.

In the United States, health-care costs now total $3.2 trillion a year, accounting for nearly 18 percent of our gross domestic product. Poor health is good business for pharmaceutical companies and hospitals: We take pills to deal with high blood pressure, high cholesterol, blood sugar imbalance, chronic pain, and countless other maladies. We undergo test after test to figure out why our bodies are out of whack. We subject ourselves to invasive surgeries to clear out masses and reroute arteries. We try to fix everything except our dinner plates.

What if there was a better way? What if we could get all the protein we needed without having to worry about it destroying our health? What if Mark could attain the physique he wanted without overdosing on animal protein and taxing his heart? What if Samantha could lose excess weight naturally and safely, and keep it off for life? What if Sally could finally sleep easily knowing that her daughter is receiving all the healthy protein a growing girl needs?

The answer is not less protein, although that's part of it, too. The answer is *clean* protein.

Think about how the nation is switching to hybrids and fully electric cars to reduce our reliance on dirty fossil fuel energy.

You get the same performance, only cleaner. It's cheaper in that you don't have to buy so much (if any) gasoline, and it's better for the environment. In that same vein, think about experiencing all the benefits that so many protein enthusiasts attribute to their high-protein diet—stronger muscles, healthy hair, glowing skin—without any of the heart disease, diabetes, and increased cancer risk. Same protein performance, but cleaner.

As Americans, we are accustomed to heaps of protein at the center of our plate. That's the way we are, and that isn't likely to change. But imagine if you could effortlessly switch to protein that is healthy, sustainable, inexpensive, and just as delicious.

Now imagine doing this all *today*.

This is the clean protein revolution, and it's beginning in kitchens and at dinner tables around the country. It's beginning with families who are ridding themselves of medical bills and drugs. It's beginning with children who are growing up strong and lean and healthy. It's beginning with seniors who are living comfortably into their advanced years.

It's beginning with you, right now.

PART 1

The Truth About Protein

CHAPTER 1

What, Why, and How Much?

Sure, everyone has heard of protein. But what it is exactly? Everyone agrees that it's vital, but, for some, protein means big muscles. For others, protein means energy. Many think that protein means meat. Because protein is the most sacred, celebrated, and misunderstood of all the nutrients, it means a lot of things to a lot of people. So let's clear up the confusion.

Put simply, protein means *life*. It is one of six nutrients that are essential for your body to function, the others being water, vitamins, minerals, carbohydrates, and fat. Protein is the building block of life. Just as bricks and mortar form the foundation of a house, protein forms the physical structure of your body and is critical to facilitating growth and development, repairing damage, and keeping you functioning.

Protein itself is composed of twenty smaller building blocks called amino acids, eleven of which your body creates on its own; these are called nonessential amino acids. Your body cannot synthesize nine "essential" amino acids, so you must obtain them from food. When you eat protein, your digestive system breaks it down into amino acids, which are then dispatched to build and repair cells, bones, teeth, skin—anything your body needs.

Protein is critical to your immune response and eliminating unhealthy cells, while proteins called antibodies attack viruses directly and stimulate the natural killer cells that seek and destroy cancer cells. Insulin and growth hormones, which are essential to regulating sugar levels and helping young children grow, are also made up of protein. Meanwhile, all of the key neurotransmitters that regulate your emotions are derived from protein. For example, the famous mood and concentration boosters dopamine and serotonin are synthesized from the amino acids tyrosine and tryptophan, respectively. Put simply, every emotion, every feeling, every thought that passes through your mind is brought to you by protein.

Life cannot happen without protein. But, in our "if some is good, more must be better" culture, this translates as, "Eat as much protein as humanly possible." Every day we are inundated with advertisements claiming that sculpted muscles, six-pack abs, toned thighs, and size-zero dresses are just a protein shake away. If you talk with bodybuilders, you might think that protein is the only nutrient worth consuming. If you walk into any health store, you'll see tubs of protein powder with labels featuring muscular models, while brands like Muscle Milk and Pure Protein strive to outdo each other by cramming more and more protein into their products. Given all the products and misleading advertising, a reasonable person might think there is a protein deficiency epidemic in the United States and around the world. However, if anything, we have the opposite problem. The diseases that plague Americans, as we will discuss more in the next chapter, have to do with too *much* consumption rather than too *little*.

HOW MUCH PROTEIN DO WE NEED?

The answers to this question can be confusing, and there is a lot of bad information out there—not just on the Internet, but also in books, magazines, and even reputable newspapers. With a little digging, however, the answer is actually quite clear. According to the National Academy of Medicine, the current and best recommendation for protein intake is approximately 0.8 grams per kilogram of healthy body weight per day. This includes an err-on-the-side-of-caution buffer, so most people actually require less. When we say "healthy body weight," that means that if you weigh 220 pounds but your healthy body weight is 175, you calculate your protein needs based on 175 pounds, not 220.

So a 130-pound woman should consume around 45 grams of protein, and a 180-pound man should be consuming around 65 grams. For moderately active people at those weights, caloric intake should be approximately 1,850 and 2,450 calories, respectively—this means that protein intake should be approximately 10 percent of total calories. Growing kids need a bit more protein: about 1.1 grams per kilogram of body weight. As it turns out, though, American adults and children are typically consuming about 50 percent more protein than they actually need.

As recounted by investigative journalist Marta Zaraska in her brilliant history of humankind's fixation with meat, *Meathooked*, protein obsession began in the 1820s with a German scientist named Justus von Liebig, who "glorified protein as the only real nutrient and believed that without it our muscles just wouldn't work." Unsurprisingly, the good doctor started a company to market Liebig's Extract of Meat—the Muscle Milk of its day.

Another nineteenth-century physiologist, Carl von Voit, recommended with practically no evidence that adults consume 150 grams of protein per day. After studying the protein intake of manual laborers, von Voit simply extrapolated that amount to arrive at his recommendation for average adults. As Zaraska notes, von Voit's methodology was "like observing children stuffing themselves with cookies and concluding that young humans require tons of sugar to grow." Although von Voit later conceded that protein intake should be closer to 50 grams per day, his first declaration remained conventional wisdom.

Few people challenged this belief until the early twentieth century, when Yale University chemist Russell Chittenden decided to test von Voit's methodology. Chittenden is best known as the "father of American biochemistry," but we could also reasonably refer to him as the "father of protein sanity." Against great opposition Chittenden proved that humans don't need more than 10 percent of their calories from protein, and what was considered protein deficiency at the time was actually simple malnutrition from lack of caloric intake.

Chittenden arrived at his recommendations after reviewing all of the scientific research on human protein needs. He was surprised by the lack of any evidence to support high-protein diets. Intrigued, he decided to drastically cut protein from his own diet and even convinced his friends and family to do the same. Chittenden figured that if von Voit's protein recommendations were accurate, he and his subjects would be weaker, have worse concentration, and exhibit lower productivity. On the contrary, their health and alertness improved markedly.

Then, beginning in 1903, Chittenden organized experiments over a six-month period with military men who were beginning their training. These men were accustomed to eating very large quantities of meat, so Chittenden reduced their meat intake by about two-thirds. He also subjected them to fifteen strength and fitness tests. After he slashed their meat intake, these men, who were already quite fit, doubled their average fitness scores. He then repeated the experiment with well-trained athletes, who, just as the military men, were accustomed to high meat intake. Once again, the participants' performance improved—this time by about 35 percent.

By the 1940s, the USDA protein recommendations were a reasonable 70 grams per day for men and 60 for women—still high, but a fraction of what was recommended by the protein-crazed nineteenth-century Germans. Nevertheless, the protein myth was reborn with a poorly designed study involving rats. The authors claimed—without any evidence at all—that protein needs for rats were the same as for humans. This makes no sense, because rats are natural carnivores and rat babies grow extremely quickly compared to human babies, while rat milk contains nearly four times more protein than does human milk. Alas, we are not rats. And in general, as long as we are getting enough calories, we are getting enough protein.

WHICH PROTEIN IS BEST?

As we will see in this book, just about *every whole food has protein,* from sirloin steaks to iceberg lettuce to lentils to oranges. For this reason, protein deficiency is extraordinarily rare in the United States. While animal products are the most concentrated sources of protein, people who don't eat meat, eggs, and dairy still meet the protein recommendation with ease. A study published in the *Journal of the Academy of Nutrition and Dietetics* comprising 30,000 meat-eaters and 25,000 non-meat-eaters found that every participant who was consuming adequate calories received enough protein, with even the strictest plant-based eaters receiving 70 percent more protein than they needed.

In short, if you aren't drastically underweight, then you are receiving enough protein in your diet, no matter what you are eating. Nevertheless, the animal-food industry is desperate to convince Americans that they need more, more, more protein and that meat is the best source. With revenues exceeding $250 billion and an annual advertising budget in the hundreds of millions, the industry can afford to perpetuate this myth indefinitely. Read that again, if you will: revenues for animal protein exceed $250 billion per year. Marketing campaigns such as "Got Milk?" and "Beef. It's What's for Dinner," have convinced millions that animal protein is a normal, healthy, and essential part of their diet. The acclaimed investigative journalist Upton Sinclair famously observed, "It is difficult to get a man to understand something, when his salary depends on his not understanding it." Executives for the American Meat Institute and the National Chicken Council are paid to believe that everyone should eat more beef and chicken, and so it's sound business practice to spend vast sums convincing people they will waste away from protein deficiency without animal products.

OK, you might be thinking. *So we're eating more protein than we need. What's the big deal?*

Most pressingly, all of those extra calories are leading to extreme weight gain. A study funded by the Bill and Melinda Gates Foundation and published in the *Lancet* reports that obesity rates have been rising over the past three decades globally—so much so that roughly 40 percent of the global population is now either overweight or obese. In short, obesity now presents "a major public health epidemic in both the developed and the developing world." As the authors conclude, "In the last three decades, not one country has achieved success in reducing obesity rates, and we expect obesity to rise steadily as incomes rise in low- and middle-income countries in particular, unless urgent steps are taken to address this public health crisis." Ironically, according to the food market research firm Mintel, two-thirds of consumers believe that eating high-protein foods is the best way to lose weight.

Major news stories about obesity epidemics are as common as stories about heart disease, cancer, and diabetes—each of which is linked to being overweight. In contrast, when was the last time you read a story about a protein deficiency epidemic? You will not find such an article, because not only is there no protein deficiency epidemic, there is no protein deficiency at all. Period.

But this book is not about how to eat less protein, because protein is not actually the culprit—the culprit is animal protein. So this book is about how to eat *better* protein. If so many foods can provide you with ample amounts of protein, then which do you eat? It turns out there are vast differences in quality among various forms of protein. Some protein you can eat to your heart's content, and your body will remain happy—this is what we refer to as *clean protein*. Other forms of protein are fine in small amounts but can cause serious disease when consumed regularly—we call this *dirty protein*. In the next chapter we will break down these differences.

CHAPTER 2

The Ideal Source

The doctor of the future will no longer treat the human frame with drugs, but rather will cure and prevent disease with nutrition.

—Thomas Edison

In 2008, the Westland/Hallmark Meat Packing Company made a stunning announcement: They were ordering a recall of a record 143 million pounds of beef, many of it used for school lunches. This was the equivalent of two hamburgers for every man, woman, and child in the United States. The recall dwarfed the previous record, set in 1999, when 35 million pounds of beef potentially contaminated with listeria were removed from store shelves. Westland/Hallmark was forced to issue the massive recall after undercover footage by the Humane Society revealed workers beating cows and illegally using forklifts to force sick cows to walk. The meat from cows who cannot walk, known as "downers," may be tainted with human-transferable pathogens, most notably mad cow disease.

Three years later, in 2011, a drug-resistant strain of salmonella sickened seventy-six people and killed one in twenty-six states. The outbreak was traced to a Cargill Meat Solutions plant in Arkansas, and the company voluntarily recalled 36 million pounds of ground turkey—more than the weight of thirty-six fully-loaded Boeing 747 jumbo jets.

While meat contamination of this particular sort is relatively rare, these stories accentuate one of the biggest problems with eating animals: Because their flesh contains a high percentage of fat, they harbor toxins and dangerous bacteria long after slaughter. Whether it's heavy metals in fish or E. coli in beef, animal protein is the most prolific cause of foodborne illness among humans. But there's more . . .

For many Americans, meat is protein and protein is meat. They see no distinction. Both of the authors of this book are plant based, and we are frequently asked, "How do you get your protein?"—as if only meat, dairy, and eggs contain this vital nutrient. We politely explain that meat is not the only, or even the best, source of protein, in large part because animal protein consumption is linked to a wide variety of serious health problems.

Dr. Garth Davis, author of the superb book *Proteinaholic*, sums up the case against animal protein by noting that the people who eat the most animal protein globally are "the most overweight and sick populations." Indeed, the peer-reviewed journal *Nutrition* reviewed thirty-two studies—twenty-one clinical and eleven reviews—and found that high meat intake is clearly associated with bone deterioration, kidney disorders, increased cancer risk, liver disease, and heart disease. The authors conclude "that there is currently no reasonable scientific basis in the literature to recommend protein consumption above the current [Recommended Daily Allowance] for healthy adults due to its potential disease risks." Meanwhile, the Johns Hopkins Bloomberg School of Public

Health declares that "a strong body of scientific evidence links excess meat consumption with heart disease, stroke, type 2 diabetes, obesity, certain cancers, and earlier death." The National Academy of Sciences published a paper in 2016 that finds that a "shift away from meat consumption could cut premature mortality globally by 6–10 percent."

Animal protein consumption is linked to a wide range of serious health problems, though it's not clear whether the cause is animal protein itself or other components in meat, such as saturated fat. Heart researcher and founder of the Preventive Medicine Research Institute, Dr. Dean Ornish, notes in the *New York Times*, "Research shows that animal protein may significantly increase the risk of premature mortality from all causes, among them cardiovascular disease, cancer and type II diabetes. Heavy consumption of saturated fat and trans fats may double the risk of developing Alzheimer's disease."

In other words, using meat as your primary protein delivery mechanism turns out to be exceedingly risky. Animal product consumption is linked to an array of chronic diseases, including heart disease, obesity, cancer, diabetes, Alzheimer's, bone deterioration, and impotence. Let's touch on each briefly.

HEART DISEASE

Heart disease is the number one killer in the developed world. In the United States, it is responsible for 25 percent of all deaths, or more than 600,000 each year. This is a remarkable statistic considering nearly every one of these deaths could be easily prevented.

Remember Mark from earlier in the book, who was wolfing down protein to improve his physique? As his doctor discovered, that 190 grams per day of protein isn't just going to his pecs—it's also going to his heart.

According to the Physicians Committee for Responsible Medicine (PCRM), which has done an extensive review of the literature covering disease prevention, heart disease "can be virtually eliminated by controlling three factors: cholesterol, smoking, and blood pressure." PCRM notes that cutting meat out of your diet "may be nearly as effective as some cholesterol-reducing medications." Up until thirty years ago, there was a scientific consensus that heart disease and old age were inextricably linked. As you got older, if you didn't get hit by a bus or a falling piano, eventually your arteries would clog up naturally and stop your heart. Heart disease was considered as inevitable as middle-aged myopia. Dr. Ornish was not convinced. After putting his patients on a low-fat, plant-based diet combined with lifestyle changes like exercise and meditation, he not only stopped the progression of their heart disease but reversed it entirely.

A few years later, Dr. Caldwell Esselstyn from the Cleveland Clinic replicated Ornish's results with a plant-based diet as the only lifestyle intervention. Once again, patients with extreme heart disease managed to completely reverse their prognosis. Dr. Esselstyn explains, "Anyone who follows the program faithfully will almost certainly see no further progression of disease, and will very likely find that it selectively regresses. And the corollary, overwhelmingly supported by global population studies, is that persons without the disease who adopt these same dietary changes will never develop heart disease."

CANCER

Cancer is the number two killer in the developed world and may soon overtake heart disease for the top spot. The average American male has an almost 50 percent chance of developing cancer at some point in his life, and the average woman has an almost 40 percent chance. And the data suggest the risk will continue to increase.

As with heart disease, cancer is largely preventable. For example, many scientists believe that as many as four-fifths of breast and prostate cancer diagnoses are a result of poor diet, and studies clearly show that excess animal product consumption is a leading culprit. That's why the American Institute for Cancer Research declares without equivocation, "When it comes to American health, the research shows one thing very clearly: We all need to eat more plants and less meat."

Poultry consumption in particular is closely associated with the progression of prostate cancer. One study of 27,000 men published in the journal *Cancer Prevention Research* finds a 69 percent greater risk of lethal prostate cancer among men who consumed 3.5 or more servings of poultry weekly compared with those who consumed fewer than 2 servings per week. An extra 1.5 servings—which is just two pieces of chicken per week—increased cancer risk by almost 70 percent. Researchers speculate that the culprit might be heterocyclic amines (HCAs), toxic compounds that form when animal protein is subjected to high heat (e.g., grilling, broiling, or frying). HCAs are linked to many forms of cancer including breast, colon, liver, skin, lung, and prostate cancer.

But the problem isn't just with HCAs. Animal protein is extremely potent and helps fuel the excessive growth of human cells. Much of that growth potential is directed toward the only cells that crave more fuel: cancer cells. Dr. Walter Willett, chair of the Department of Nutrition at Harvard's School of Public Health, explains that "animal protein . . . tends to make cells multiply faster. . . . This is one of the fundamental processes that increase the risk of cancer." Indeed, an analysis cited by the Academy of Nutrition and Dietetics finds that vegetarians have an almost 20 percent lower risk of contracting cancer when compared to people who include meat in their diets.

That's a conservative figure; the real numbers may be much higher. For example, a 2014 study in the journal *Cell Metabolism* finds that the more animal protein people eat during middle age, the more likely they are to succumb to cancer. "Respondents aged 50 to 65 reporting high protein intake had a 75% increase in overall mortality and a 4-fold increase in cancer death risk during the following 18 years," the study notes. "These associations were either abolished or attenuated if the proteins were plant derived."

In a press release, University of Southern California director of research communications Suzanne Wu explains, "That chicken wing you're eating could be as deadly as a cigarette. In a new study that tracked a large sample of adults for nearly two decades, researchers have found that eating a diet rich in animal proteins during middle age makes you four times more likely to die of cancer than someone with a low-protein diet—a mortality risk factor comparable to smoking."

OBESITY

Obesity levels in the developed world have reached epidemic proportions. Universally considered to be a preventable disease, obesity is a leading cause of death worldwide. Obesity may not directly cause heart disease, cancer, or diabetes, but those who are obese are far more likely to be eating a diet associated with these diseases.

During his heart disease studies, Dr. Ornish found that in addition to unclogging his patients' arteries and curing their chest pain (angina), they also had more energy, felt better, lost weight—and kept it off. Consistently, lower meat consumption has been associated with a healthy weight, which is why the Academy of Nutrition and Dietetics tells its members they "should be aware of the evidence to support the use of vegetarian and vegan diets for achieving and maintaining a healthy weight." The academy cites multiple studies, all of which indicate that the more animal products people consume, the higher their likelihood of being overweight or obese.

How Your Body Reacts to One Fat-Heavy Meal

Dr. Dean Ornish has converted countless patients to a clean protein diet largely by explaining to them the effect of a single high-saturated-fat meal. Here is what happens:

First, the saturated fat in products like milk, butter, and meat causes your blood to thicken with liquid fat, reducing blood flow to the heart and everywhere else. This contributes to the angina and general achiness that many heart disease patients feel after a big meal.

Second, your arteries stiffen. Saturated fat triggers what Ornish calls endothelial dysfunction, which means your arteries constrict and grow stiffer. Among healthy people, arteries are supple and flexible, so they can adapt to a fatty meal once in a while. But a lifetime of dirty protein makes your arteries hard and brittle, so a single fatty meal can further slow blood flow.

Third, a fatty meal promotes plaque buildup—the precursor to coronary heart disease. The more fat and LDL (bad) cholesterol in your blood, the more waxy plaque that accumulates in your arteries. A study published in the *Journal of the American College of Cardiology* proves how a single high-fat meal reduces the anti-inflammatory ability of HDL (good) cholesterol to protect your artery lining from plaque buildup.

Finally, a fatty meal leads to what Ornish calls the "Holiday Effect," the sad tendency for heart attacks to occur during the holiday season, when people consume more high-fat foods. A single meal high in saturated fat can decrease blood flow so significantly that, for too many people, the first symptom of heart disease can also be the last.

So it raises the question: Are bacon and eggs really worth the risk?

Generally, people who avoid meat entirely are about half as likely to be overweight as people who eat meat, and studies show that plant-eaters are 10 to 25 percent lighter than meat-eaters.

Remember Samantha from the introduction? Like so many Americans, she believes that substituting carbohydrates with high-protein animal products could help her lose weight. At first the weight can indeed come off as long as a high-protein diet is accompanied by calorie restriction. But that weight loss often doesn't last. Depriving yourself of calories rarely works long-term, because it's unsustainable. If you're eating eggs and bacon and little else, you'll likely feel unsatisfied, long-term. But if you're eating healthy, unrefined plant protein that the brain and body actually need and therefore crave, you'll feel satisfied; the abundant fiber from the whole grains, beans, nuts, and fruits will fill you up and keep you steady.

DIABETES

Diabetes is a disease in which your body cannot properly process food for use as energy. A hormone called insulin normally helps shuttle energy, known as glucose (basically sugar), to your cells. But, among diabetics, this process is impaired either because insulin production is insufficient or because their cells won't accept it, leading to dangerously high levels of glucose in the blood.

Some people are born with this condition and must have insulin injections for life—this is called type 1 diabetes. But by far the more common form of diabetes is type 2 diabetes, formerly known as adult-onset diabetes. Type 2 diabetes goes hand in hand with obesity: roughly 90 percent of diabetics are obese. So it's not surprising that diabetes incidence has exploded in almost perfect alignment with obesity, with almost four times more type 2 diabetics today than in the early 1980s.

While there is a clear link between obesity and type 2 diabetes, simply eating meat can increase your risk even if you are not obese. According to the Adventists health studies, which followed tens of thousands of predominantly plant-based Christians known as Seventh-Day Adventists, there is a linear relationship between animal product consumption and diabetes. Complete vegans are 62 percent less likely to develop diabetes when compared to meat-eaters, and vegetarians are almost 40 percent less likely to contract the disease.

If you have diabetes, simply cutting out animal products can reverse the disease entirely. In one study, diabetic patients who switched to a diet centered on whole plant foods were able to stop taking nearly all their medications after their blood markers dropped to nondiabetic levels.

ALZHEIMER'S

Alzheimer's is perhaps the most dreaded disease. It's often referred to as "the long goodbye" because it destroys victims' minds one memory at a time, eventually reducing a grown adult's faculties to those of a toddler. While Alzheimer's is the sixth leading killer in the United States, having claimed almost 100,000 lives in 2015, the Alzheimer's Association notes that it is the third leading cause of death of older adults, after heart disease and cancer.

Alzheimer's rates are rising worldwide, and there is extensive evidence linking it to animal protein consumption. For example, a metareview published in the *Journal of the American College of Nutrition* finds that nothing is more predictive of Alzheimer's than diet; as just one example, rates of Alzheimer's in Japan grew by a staggering 700 percent after the Japanese shifted toward a Western diet beginning in the mid-1980s. The authors conclude that "reducing meat consumption could significantly reduce the risk of

[Alzheimer's Disease] as well as of several cancers, diabetes mellitus type 2, stroke, and, likely, chronic kidney disease."

Large population studies also suggest that a plant-based diet is protective against Alzheimer's disease. Rural India, whose population subsists mainly on grains, legumes, and vegetables, has the lowest documented rates of Alzheimer's in the world.

BONE DETERIORATION

The word "osteoporosis" comes from the Greek words *osteo*, meaning "bone," and *poro*, meaning "porous." Add "sis," and you've got a disease. So, porous-bone disease—that pretty much sums it up. People who suffer from osteoporosis have bones that become brittle from loss of tissue. They can fracture and break from falls—or even bumps and sneezes. According to the International Osteoporosis Foundation, porous bones lead to hip, wrist, and other fractures almost 9 million times per year globally, with more than half of these cases in the United States and Europe.

Ironically, milk consumption—which the milk industry wants us to believe is good for our bones—appears to actually increase risk of bone fractures. Researchers writing in the *Journal of Bone and Mineral Research* looked at all the best studies and find no indication that milk consumption is good for our bones, even as many studies show that a higher rate of milk intake is associated with higher rates of bone fracture.

For example, a set of studies published in the *BMJ* followed 100,000 people for two decades and finds that milk can actually *increase* the rates of bone and hip fractures in women, contrary to what all those "Milk Does a Body Good" ads might suggest.

Studies also indicate that substituting plant protein for animal protein can decrease fracture risk. Notably, increased calcium consumption does not seem to help. However, resistance exercises can help strengthen bones, just as it can with your muscles.

IMPOTENCE

Clogged arteries don't just mean decreased blood flow to your heart—it means decreased blood flow *everywhere*. If clogged arteries can lead to heart disease and Alzheimer's disease, they can also lead to impotence. Approximately 1 in 10 men over the age of forty has severe or complete erectile dysfunction—a problem that only increases with age and can even begin during the teen years. One study finds that two-thirds of men suffering from severe heart disease also experienced impotence. In fact, erectile dysfunction pills such as Viagra work very similarly to angina medication—by dilating arteries to improve blood flow. That's because heart disease and erectile dysfunction are effectively the same condition.

It's ironic how polls consistently show that men are far more likely to feel that eating less meat will somehow damage their manhood. In fact, the opposite is true. Another outcome of Dr. Ornish's work is his discovery that blood flow to his patients' hearts improved 300 percent, restoring sexual function in men and pleasure for their partners. Of course, the fact that episodes of chest pain decreased by more than 90 percent within a few weeks also lowered the risk of patients having a heart attack while engaged in sexual activity—and it's hard to imagine something less manly than that.

WHAT ABOUT FISH?

All of the diseases we discussed appear to be linked to either the saturated fat or the protein in animal foods. What about fish consumption, which is generally seen as healthier than other meats? Actually, besides its saturated fat, fish has a major problem: toxins. It turns out the heavy metals found in many fish can lead to cognitive problems, a problem so common it has its own nickname: "fish fog."

"Waiter, is that mercury in my sushi?"

If your sushi is made with fish, the answer is quite likely yes. The *New York Times* bought and tested tuna sushi from twenty Manhattan grocery stores and restaurants, finding that many were tainted with high levels of mercury, a poison that humans consume almost exclusively from fish, according to the EPA, which can cause brain damage, memory loss, tremors, and joint pain. If you want to be turned off fish forever, read *Diagnosis Mercury: Money, Politics, and Poison,* by Dr. Jane Hightower.

Hightower was confused when many of her patients complained of hair loss, fatigue, depression, difficulty concentrating, and headaches. When she finally took her patients off fish, their symptoms disappeared. The *Wall Street Journal* ran a front-page story about one of Dr. Hightower's patients, a preteen named Matthew Davis. Matthew went from being an honors student and playing sports to struggling with his schoolwork and being unable to catch a football. Once Matthew stopped eating canned tuna, his symptoms disappeared.

A study in the journal *Science Advances* found in 2017 that, as land use and coastal temperatures increase, organic matter runoff will increase by 10 to 50 percent. This can lead to mercury concentrations that are 200 to 700 percent greater than the already highly toxic concentrations currently present in fish. The Environmental Defense Fund points out that mercury is not the only toxin that can build up in fish flesh: "Fish can also absorb organic chemicals (such as PCBs, dioxins and DDT) from the water, suspended sediments, and their food."

Think about it this way: Would you stick a cup into the lake, river, stream, or ocean that your fish was pulled out of and drink that water? Doubtful. Yet many of the toxins in that water collect in the flesh of that fish and we, of course, consume those toxins when we eat the fish.

Why Dairy Doesn't Cut It for "Clean"

Yes, **dairy has** a good bit of protein, but you have to consider the whole picture. Here's the dirt:

1. **Cancer:** Consumption of cow's milk products has been linked to higher rates of prostate and breast cancer, likely because of the increase in IGF-1 (insulin-like growth factor) found in dairy. The estrogen metabolites can cause cells to grow quickly and aberrantly, leading to cancer growth.

2. **Lactose intolerance:** It may not sound like a big deal, but the symptoms are pretty odious: flatulence, bloating, and diarrhea.

3. **Bad bone health:** Despite the "milk is good for your bones" campaign, clinical research has shown that dairy has little or no benefit for bones and doesn't reduce fracture risk. This all applies to kids, too.

4. **Skin problems:** Dermatologists routinely recommend eliminating dairy to combat acne, especially in young people. There's increasing evidence of a correlation between a dairy-rich diet and skin breakouts.

5. **Fat and cholesterol:** Dairy is high in both, which increase the risk of heart disease. Dairy is also associated with weight gain. (Skim and low-fat milk are actually tied to more weight gain than full-fat milk.)

6. **Gross stuff:** Raw milk is sometimes contaminated with dangerous pathogens and pus from an udder infection called mastitis that cows get from near-constant milk production.

FAT: GOOD OR BAD,
AND ARE WE EATING MORE OF IT?

There is a common and false narrative that runs like this: In the 1970s we were all told that saturated fat was the devil and we should eat less of it. We ate less of it, and we got fatter. Ergo, saturated fat is not the enemy.

This narrative, extremely convenient for the meat industry and anyone who loves fast food, is dangerously wrong. As we will discuss more in Chapter 6, unsaturated fats, like those found in nuts, are actually healthy. But much of the fat in American diets is saturated—fat that is solid at room temperature—and that is the source of the controversy. And although there has been some debate in the popular press about whether animal products and high levels of saturated fat are bad for human health, the science is clear.

According to the USDA, total meat consumption in the 1950s was roughly 140 pounds per year. In the 1970s, it was 177 pounds per year. That figure went up in the '80s, up again in the '90s, and by the 2000s was nearly 200 pounds. Americans have steadily consumed more meat, more saturated fat, more calories, and we have become progressively sicker. Nutritionists remain flummoxed by diets like Atkins, which claim bacon and eggs can be used to lose weight and that eating pasta and rice will make you fat.

In fact, studies routinely show that the slimmest people in the world are eating rice and pasta with very little meat, while the fattest people in the world are eating lots of meat and cheese with little rice or pasta. When people in the developing world begin eating more like us, they get fatter and unhealthier. When people in the West eat a more plant-based diet, they inevitably slim down. Sensationalist stories in the media do feature studies in which participants were successful using high-protein diets, but these gimmicks are always very short term and require severe, unsustainable caloric restriction.

And, sure enough, the science backs what common sense and elementary observation indicate. In his groundbreaking work *The China Study*, Dr. T. Colin Campbell points out what many others before and since have noted: No long-term study has ever demonstrated sustained weight loss on a high-protein, high-meat diet. The only diet that has ever allowed people to lose weight and keep it off is a low-saturated-fat diet with few—and ideally zero—animal products. In one study discussed by Dr. Campbell, participants who consumed a very low-calorie diet lost weight. Yet that was not sustainable, and the side effects included constipation, bad breath, headache, hair loss, and excessive urinary calcium loss, which is a predictable effect of eating a lot of animal protein. And, after five years, most of the people who went on these diets ended up fatter compared to when they began the diet. As Dr. Campbell quips, "You can also lose weight by undergoing chemotherapy or starting a heroin addiction, but I wouldn't recommend those, either."

CHAPTER 3

The Trashing

The world is groaning under the weight of animal agriculture, and the ill effects of animal protein are not just limited to your health. From deforestation to climate change to ocean depletion, we are on a collision course with global calamity—all because of our choices at the dinner table.

CHICKEN AND THE ENVIRONMENT

In the United States, 9 billion chickens are slaughtered every year. Think for a moment about the sheer amount of feed required to raise so many birds at that scale. In fact, only a small fraction of what is fed to a chicken—or a cow or pig, for that matter—is actually converted into meat; most of it is burned off to keep the animal alive, and more than half of the food calories create skin, blood, feathers, and other inedible parts of the animal.

According to the World Resources Institute, "Even poultry, the most efficient source of meat, convert only around 11 percent of gross feed energy into human food according to the most comprehensive [scientific] methods." So you need to feed a chicken 9 calories to get 1 calorie from the animal's flesh at slaughter. Put another way, in order to sustain yourself on 2,000 calories of plant-based foods, you simply eat 2,000 calories. However, if you want to sustain yourself on 2,000 calories of chicken, you first need 18,000 calories of animal feed. These numbers are even worse for turkey, pork, and beef.

On October 5, 1947, the *New York Times* ran a front-page story entitled, "Truman Calls on Nation to Forego Meat Tuesdays, Poultry, Eggs Thursdays." President Truman was making the very basic point that meat is a highly inefficient food source, one that drove up prices and promoted widespread hunger. The *Times* reported, "Food from the United States . . . would deter the march of hunger, cold and collapse, not only enabling Europe to recover its economic stability, but also contributing to the resolution of a crisis that could mean the difference between the failure or attainment of world peace and security."

The Worldwatch Institute explains that "grain is used more efficiently when consumed directly by humans. Continued growth in meat output is dependent on feeding grain to animals, creating competition for grain between affluent meat eaters and the world's poor." And Oxfam America writes, "Eating less meat is a simple way to reduce the pressure on global resources and help ensure that everyone has enough to eat. To say it simply, eating less meat helps fight hunger."

Of course, nine times as many crops means nine times as much pesticide and nine times as much water. But that's not all. Think about the extra stages of production: You have to grow the feed crops, ship the crops to a feed mill, operate the feed mill, ship the feed to the farm, operate the farm, ship the animals to the slaughterhouse, operate the slaughterhouse, ship the meat to a processor, and so on. Every stage involves both significant energy requirements and significant pollution. Scientists from the United Nations crunched the numbers and determined that the meat industry is responsible for more climate change than all forms of transportation combined, as well as "problems of land degradation and air pollution, water shortage and water pollution and loss of biodiversity."

On the issue of climate change, chicken is the least climate change–inducing meat, and yet *Environment* magazine reports that chicken creates forty times as much climate change per protein calorie when compared to legumes such as peas and soy (the most common ingredients in plant-based meat). Researchers at the Royal Institute of International Affairs, more commonly referred to as Chatham House, have reviewed all of the scientific literature on the contributions of animal agriculture to climate change and argue that it will be impossible for countries to meet their obligation under the Paris Agreement to keep climate change under 2°C by 2050 unless animal protein consumption decreases dramatically. While animal protein consumption in the developed world has plateaued, consumption in the developing world is going up.

THE END OF WORKING ANTIBIOTICS

The animal agriculture industry in the United States uses approximately 70 percent of all "medically important" antibiotics, so if you are eating nonorganic meat, you are eating animals who were treated with antibiotics. The meat industry uses these drugs to keep animals alive in filthy conditions and to make them grow quickly for less cost. The poultry industry is most culpable, because birds receive more antibiotics than pigs or cattle do.

Farm animals are fed many of the same antibiotics that humans receive for urinary tract infections, pneumonia, and other ailments. With so many animals living in unsanitary conditions, experts warn that dangerous pathogens may evolve and become resistant to antibiotics. That means that when we get sick or have an infection and need antibiotics, those antibiotics won't work. This was once rare, but so-called superbugs are increasingly able to thwart every known antibiotic. The more antibiotics that meat producers use, the higher the risk of resistant superbugs infecting humans. Dr. Margaret Chen, director-general of the World Health Organization (WHO), warns, "A post-antibiotic era means, in effect, an end to modern medicine as we know it. Things as common as strep throat or a child's scratched knee could once again kill."

An investigation by Reuters finds that all of the major poultry producers in the country were using antibiotics in their animals. And a recent story on National Public Radio reports that a Nevada woman died of an incurable infection "resistant to all 26 antibiotics available in the U.S." The Centers for Disease Control and Prevention notes that 23,000 Americans die each year from infections that are resistant to one or more antibiotics.

Tom Philpott of *Mother Jones* sums it up this way:

> Currently, livestock operations burn through about 70 percent of the "medically important" antibiotics used in the nation—the ones people need when an infection strikes. Microbes that have evolved to withstand antibiotics now sicken 2 million Americans each year and kill 23,000 others—more than homicide. Even though public health authorities from the Food and Drug Administration and the Centers for Disease Control and Prevention have long pointed to the meat industry's reliance on antibiotics as a major culprit in human resistance to the drugs, the FDA has never reined in their use.

Remarkably, nonorganically raised animals are also fed a variety of other chemicals. Research from Johns Hopkins University found caffeine, diphenhydramine (the active antihistamine in Benadryl), acetaminophen (the active ingredient of Tylenol), the antidepressant Prozac, and arsenic in poultry. According to *New*

York Times journalist Nicholas Kristof, these drugs are given to reduce anxiety, and, in the case of caffeine, to increase eating and thus weight. Kristof quips, "Frankly, after reading these studies, I'm so depressed about what has happened to farming that I wonder: Could a Prozac-laced chicken nugget help?"

FISH AND THE DEATH OF AQUATIC ECOSYSTEMS

The old adage is wrong: there are not plenty of fish in the sea. In fact, although technology is good for many things, environmental preservation is not one of them. The adverse environmental impact of fishing may be less obvious, because most people haven't seen firsthand the practices that are involved in catching tuna, salmon, and shrimp. Whether we're looking at commercial fishing or fish farming, the external environmental costs of fish consumption rival those of terrestrial agriculture.

Where it may well have been true years ago that humans could not catch more fish than could be replenished, those days are long past. By weight, commercial fishers are pillaging our aquatic ecosystems to the tune of 1 to 2 billion metric tons per year, according to an estimate in the journal *Science,* which is many times what our oceans can replenish. As a result, most of our world's fisheries are depleted or in decline.

Fishing also wreaks havoc on aquatic ecosystems. For example, clams are harvested by dredging along the water bed, which depletes oxygen and kills other sea life. Similarly, commercial trawlers drag football field–sized nets along the seafloor, snagging and killing their target catch along with countless other creatures including oysters, which serve as important filters of nitrogen and phosphates. With too much of these nutrients in the water, entire ecosystems can die off.

Other problems include abandoned fishing gear that kills fish and birds and poisons waterways. Fishing boats can be so indiscriminate that there is a term—"bycatch"—for the enormous amount of nontarget species that are caught in fishing nets. Longline fishing, meanwhile, involves fishing boats dragging miles-long lines containing thousands of baited hooks. Fish such as tuna and swordfish are then dragged behind the boat until they either die or become exhausted from a lack of oxygen. Every year, longliners also claim the lives of hundreds of thousands of bycatch animals, including birds, sharks, dolphins, and turtles.

Not all fish are caught in the wild. More and more, fish are raised on massive fish farms, which present an array of potential ecological problems. For example, fish grown and genetically bred for bulk on farms can escape into natural ecosystems. This can lead to genetic degradation of wild animals and the introduction of disease or parasites. Commercially farmed fish tend to grow more quickly because of their incredibly high-protein feed, all of the growth-promoting drugs they are fed, and their lethargic daily life that involves little other than eating, so they will have much weaker immune systems. Many fish farms are simply large cages in oceans and lakes, which can be susceptible to rupture. Farmed fish that escape and breed with their wild counterparts can cause a complete population collapse.

Many fish farms are adjacent to natural waterways and crammed with an unfathomable number of fish. Most of the fish would die in these atrocious conditions if fish farmers did not use enormous quantities of antibiotics. These drugs, along with the unnatural amount of fish waste, can easily escape into the surrounding ecosystem, polluting aquatic ecosystems almost beyond recognition. One study found that salmon farming can reduce the survival rates of nearby wild populations by 50 percent or more thanks to deadly concentrations of bacteria.

There are myriad harms associated with animal protein that, in our view, qualify it as dirty protein. Private equity billionaire Jeremy Coller launched an effort to call on global food companies to diversify their protein holdings away from animals and toward plant and cellular alternatives, and he was able to get dozens of investment firms representing more than $2 trillion to join. According to Coller, the meat industry "is emerging as a high-risk production method linked with significant environmental damage and major public health issues, such as the emergence of antibiotic resistant bacteria and outbreaks of pandemics such as avian flu." Smart man, and we agree.

The world's population is rising, the demand for protein is growing, and the current system of raising animals for food is, quite simply, not sustainable. The land and water cannot bear the burden, nor can human health. Funneling crops through animals who are totally drugged up makes no sense, especially when there are better, cleaner options to feed the world. We'll explore those clean protein alternatives later in the book. But first, let's take a look at how animal protein became king.

CHAPTER 4

Follow the Money

The beef industry has worked hard to create the love
affair that Americans have with a big, juicy ribeye.
—*BEEF* MAGAZINE

By now, you likely understand how "dirty" protein can take
a toll on human health and the environment, but you may
scratch your head and wonder how the heck animal foods became
so entrenched in our daily diets if there's so much wrong with
them. A little bit here and there, sure; we get that the richness of
animal food can taste good. But it almost feels like this food has
been forced upon us, and, in many ways, it has. This chapter is
about connecting the dots and following the money—not surprisingly, both the dots and the money lead back to the animal food
industries.

Let's start by taking a stroll through the protein section of your
local grocery store. If you're lucky, there will be an abundance of
plant-based alternatives. You'll see that most of these products
speak to how closely they resemble the taste and texture of meat

or dairy. "Slow Roasted Chick'n," "Breakfast Sausage," "great buttery taste," deli slices that are hickory smoked or "bologna style," almond milk, and cashew cheese. Clearly these are meant as substitutes for chicken, pork, butter, and the like.

These products market themselves on how closely they taste like and resemble animal products. But why? Tempeh and tofu are perfectly delicious on their own. So why do we have to pretend they taste like meat? There isn't a multibillion-dollar industry devoted to walnut alternatives for people who are allergic to tree nuts, after all. Given the cruelty associated with animal food production, not to mention the staggering documentation of its negative effects on human health and the environment, why are we so obsessed with recreating the meat experience?

Despite overwhelming evidence to the contrary, the animal food industry has convinced the public that meat, eggs, fish, and dairy are not just healthy but *necessary* for a nutritious diet. Even more, as we'll see in this chapter, the federal government not only condones these myths but actively supports them with marketing campaigns and generous taxpayer subsidies. Thanks to relentless lobbying, financial contributions to supportive legislators, and a "revolving door" that finds regulators actually working for the industries they used to regulate, animal foods have a stranglehold on our daily diet, our tax dollars, and our public policy.

MEAT, FISH, EGGS, AND DAIRY: BROUGHT TO YOU BY THE FEDERAL GOVERNMENT

Meat producers have convinced us that we naturally crave meat, but, without extensive investments in marketing and advertising, demand for meat would be much, much lower than it is. You might have read about how this is happening with dairy in a big way: People are shunning milk products in droves, opting instead for almond-, cashew-, and soy-based alternatives. As the *Financial*

Times notes, "Worldwide sales of non-dairy milk alternatives more than doubled between 2009 and 2015 to $21 [billion]." Meanwhile, per capita consumption of traditional dairy milk plummeted by 13 percent between 2011 and 2016. During that same period, almond milk sales surged by 250 percent. As one reaction to the skyrocketing popularity of plant-based milks, Big Dairy is trying to pass legislation that would censor nondairy milk, cheese, and ice cream companies, prohibiting them from using the words "milk," "cheese," or "ice cream," to describe their products.

Swatting down healthy alternatives while promoting animal protein is a tried and true way to keep the industry robust and secure. Try randomly asking one of your neighbors, "What's for dinner?" and there's a good chance many will say, "Beef." That's largely the result of an extraordinarily successful $42 million marketing campaign by the US beef industry during the early 1990s centered around the slogan "Beef. It's What's for Dinner." You may remember some of the other slogans generated by the animal-food marketing machine including "Milk. It Does a Body Good"; "Pork. The Other White Meat"; "The Incredible, Edible Egg."

Despite study after study proving how unhealthy animal products can be, meat and egg consumption continues to rise, largely because the industry has been incredibly effective at convincing Americans that dinner is synonymous with beef, chicken, and pork, and that breakfast is synonymous with eggs. These marketing campaigns cost enormous sums of money, but the industry can easily afford them thanks to the federal government and so-called checkoff programs. Think of checkoffs as labor unions for animal food producers. Like unions, checkoffs charge mandatory dues, but, instead of helping individual workers, checkoffs help multibillion-dollar food corporations.

As instructed by Congress, $1 from every head of cattle, $0.40 from every $100 sold of pork, and $0.15 from every 100 pounds of dairy must flow to back to the industry to go toward marketing.

What's the big deal? you might be thinking. Checkoffs sound innocuous enough. Even the name "checkoff" puts you to sleep. Their bland websites feature smiling farmers and happy families. How bad can they be?

Checkoff programs were authorized by Congress with good intentions. For certain products, consumers don't care about brands, which makes advertising difficult. So instead of individual companies advertising alone, industries came together to create generic advertising to boost total demand for their products. The National Watermelon Promotion Board advertises for many different producers of watermelons, the Popcorn Board speaks on behalf of all popcorn brands, and the Christmas Tree Promotion Board . . . well, you get the point.

Checkoffs themselves aren't necessarily bad—in this case, it's the products they're selling that are bad. Because checkoffs are partnerships between the government and private industries, by law, meat, dairy, and egg companies *must* spend money to promote the consumption of animal products. Imagine if Congress passed a law guaranteeing hundreds of millions of dollars for companies to market tobacco products every single year. It's a preposterous idea, right? Yet, when you consider that at least one study found that consuming the amount of cholesterol found in just one egg per day can cut a woman's life short by as much as smoking five cigarettes daily for fifteen years, why is congressionally mandated marketing for animal food any less preposterous? It isn't, and, thanks to our elected officials, checkoff groups have a nearly $560 million annual budget for marketing disease-promoting products.

According to the USDA, Americans buy far more animal products because of checkoff marketing than they otherwise would. Without beef checkoffs, for instance, Americans would eat 11.3 percent less beef. For every $1 these organizations spend promoting their food, the return on investment can be as high as $18.

Since the beginning of "The Other White Meat" campaign in 1987, pork sales have increased by 20 percent. Dairy Management Inc., an industry group, boasted in 2011 that checkoff efforts resulted in 7 billion extra pounds of milk sold over a year and a half—that's an additional 22 pounds of milk per man, woman, and child.

Some of those checkoff dollars counter "misinformation from anti-beef groups" (we suspect, studies showing the true consequences of beef consumption), while huge sums are earmarked for influencing the most impressionable members of society: children. Checkoffs design "beef education" classes for K–12 classrooms along with marketing campaigns on social media to attract millennials. "Fuel Up to Play 60" is a campaign led by the National Football League and the National Dairy Council, which receives $50 million per year in congressionally mandated financing and influences 36 million children every year. Meanwhile, the Dairy Board checkoff has convinced 2,000 schools to provide Domino's pizza for students. The Western Dairy Association boasts that "pizza is a win for schools and for students" and that "pizza serves as a delivery vehicle for important food groups." You read that right. Pizza.

You might be thinking, *Where the heck is our government? Why are they not only allowing this, but enforcing it, and forcing it on us?* But really, why is the government involved at all?

HOW DID WE GET HERE?

In the United States, as in any country, the food supply has long been a political issue, one that's inextricable from government itself. Consider the 1928 presidential election. At a time when the average American consumed about 10 pounds of chicken per year—today we consume about 85 pounds—the Republican Party declared that Herbert Hoover would put a "chicken in every pot," and partly on the strength of that message he was elected president in a 40–8 state landslide.

Then there's the influence of the dairy industry. The government's cozy relationship with this $36 billion industry began during the Great Depression, when agricultural prices collapsed and families were losing their farms. In an effort to help farmers, the Roosevelt administration proposed and the Congress passed the Agricultural Marketing Agreement Act of 1937, allowing the federal government to set minimum prices for milk. After Congress passed the National School Lunch Act in 1946, every subsidized school lunch, by law, had to include the amount of dairy equal to a cup of whole milk. By 2009, federal nutrition programs accounted for a staggering *20 percent* of all dairy sales.

The industry grew alarmed when milk sales stagnated as Americans realized the dangers of saturated fat. A lot of us realized we were lactose intolerant or just didn't feel good when we ate cheese or drank milk. With the help of Congress and the USDA, the industry established the Dairy Checkoff in 1983 to encourage Americans to consume more milk and cheese. Thanks to a federally mandated $200 million per year budget, the Dairy Checkoff launched a marketing offensive, including the memorable "Got Milk?" campaign in 1995. Featuring celebrities and athletes in provocative poses—who can forget a shirtless, milk-mustachioed David Beckham?—"Got Milk?" was enormously successful: one study finds that in California, after years of steady decline, milk consumption jumped by 2 percent the year following the campaign's launch.

THE SHADY TRUTH BEHIND FOOD POLICY

It's not so easy to convince the government to help fund such expensive marketing campaigns. After all, you don't see Big Broccoli or Big Kale lobbyists in green suits roaming the hallways of Congress.

How does the animal food industry manage to wield such immense power?

For starters, elections help: during the 2013 election cycle, the industry contributed nearly $18 million to federal candidates and in 2014 spent almost $7 million lobbying them. As Patrick Boyle, CEO of the American Meat Institute, admits, "I think the ultimate objective of a lobbying organization such as the American Meat Institute is to be sure that when the legislators enact bills, or when a regulator finalizes a regulation, our expertise, our experience, our insight, is part of their decision-making process." Of course, the AMI's expertise, experience, and insight is going to be colored by the fact that they represent the meat industry.

It is cliché, but like so many clichés it is also true, that if you want to find out who's responsible for legislation, follow the money. That is certainly going to tell you a lot about agriculture and nutrition policy in the United States. For example, every five years the federal government releases its *Dietary Guidelines,* an enormously influential publication that determines the food served by schools, how food is labeled, how it can be marketed, and which foods can be included in assistance programs, among many other directives. Because the *Dietary Guidelines* have so much impact, food companies see their drafting as ground zero for the battle over how America eats. The Dietary Guidelines Advisory Committee drafted the initial 571-page report for 2015 based on a scientific review of thousands of studies. The report was impressively progressive: according to *Politico,* it suggested that "Americans consider both the environmental and health impacts of the food they eat" and "extolled the benefits of plant-based diets and suggested that local governments consider taxing unhealthy foods." The original guidelines advised that Americans consume "lower" amounts of red and processed meats to avoid chronic diseases such as cancer. This was very strong language from an advisory committee that, as we'll see later in this chapter, is already heavily influenced by the animal food industry. For them to advise against meat and for plant-based food, there had to be a mountain of evidence to support the recommendations—and as we know from Chapter 2, there is.

When industry groups got their hands on the draft guidelines, they promptly declared war. The American Meat Institute launched the "Hands off My Hot Dog" marketing campaign, while the National Cattlemen's Beef Association, one of the largest beef lobbying groups, spent more than $112,000 lobbying in the first three quarters of 2015 alone. Likewise, the National Pork Producers Council spent $780,000, and the North American Meat Institute threw down $220,000. The pressure worked: Department of Agriculture Secretary Tom Vilsack and Department of Health and Human Services Secretary Sylvia Mathews Burwell both assured "furious lawmakers they would steer clear of those recommendations." The finalized 2015 *Dietary Guidelines* would look nothing like the original. Instead of recommending a plant-based diet, the recommendations advocate eating "lean meats." As Marion Nestle, a food expert and nutrition professor at New York University, explains, "If I were the meat industry I would break out the champagne. Nowhere does it say eat less meat."

SUBSIDIES (HANG IN THERE—IT'S AN IMPORTANT PART OF THIS PUZZLE . . .)

While spreading misinformation is a key tactic deployed by the animal food industry, it relentlessly fights to preserve the element most crucial to its survival: taxpayer subsidies. Whereas checkoffs are primarily industry funded, subsidies mean that meat companies are supported directly by our tax dollars—whether or not you buy their products.

Public Citizen, a government watchdog group, found that congresspeople who receive money from the dairy industry are almost twice as likely to vote for dairy subsidies as those who receive no money. In a time when social programs for poor Americans endure budget cuts and outright elimination, lawmakers are eager to enlarge the bottomless, taxpayer-funded trough from which the meat, egg, and dairy industries continue to profit.

Here's an analogy: imagine that you own a car company. Unfortunately, it turns out, you're not especially adept at business because you sell your cars for less than they cost to produce. No matter the industry, if your production costs are greater than your profit, you aren't going to survive in a free-market society.

Except that for one industry, this money-losing model works perfectly well: meat. As investigative journalist and attorney David Simon calculates in his exceptional book *Meatonomics*, hog farmers routinely sell individual pigs for $8 less than they should cost to rear with open-market prices. Raising cattle makes even less business sense: a cow can sell for as much as $90 less than she costs to rear. So how does the animal-food industry make so much money? How can it survive, let alone afford such expensive lobbyists and far-reaching marketing campaigns?

Because of taxpayers like us.

Every year, taxpayers subsidize meat, fish, dairy, and egg producers to the tune of $38 billion. Without our help, most animal food producers could not create marketing campaigns to hook new generations of Americans on their products. Taxpayer subsidies even incentivize the fishing industry to maximize its catch when demand is *low*, resulting in destruction of fisheries around the globe.

While the price for most goods and services has increased along with inflation, animal food prices have actually—and artificially—*decreased*. According to the US Bureau of Labor Statistics, the inflation-adjusted price of beef fell by 53 percent between 1980 and 2008, and the price of Cheddar cheese fell by more than 26 percent. During the same period, as David Leonhardt points out in the *New York Times,* the prices of fruits and vegetables have *increased* by more than 40 percent. It's simple economics: the lower your price, the more consumers are willing to buy. The reverse is true as well: for beef, the evidence indicates that a 10 percent increase in price results in a 7.5 percent decrease in demand. According to a National Chicken Council study, 35 percent of consumers will buy more vegetables when the price of chicken increases. In short, animal food producers need to keep their prices lower than their production costs so they can continue to profit, even when it costs consumers their money and their health.

Americans are justifiably enraged when a bank requires a taxpayer bailout, but the animal food industry is effectively bailed out every single year. The backbone of these subsidies are farm bills, passed by Congress every five to seven years and designed to reduce the money factory farms spend on animal feed. This help isn't geared toward small family farmers, helping them survive so that they can eke out a living for their families; these subsidies help the massive, corporate-owned factory farms that have pushed out the little guys. Since it takes 9 calories in feed to produce 1 calorie of chicken, and even more for turkey, pork, and beef, animal food producers desperately rely on cheap grain and soy prices. According to the Global Development and Environment Institute, feed represents nearly 50 percent of the costs of raising pigs and almost two-thirds the costs of poultry and eggs.

By providing factory farming companies with a supplemental taxpayer-subsidized income, (factory) farm bills keep prices far below market value, allowing those companies to purchase artificially cheap feed. The Physicians Committee for Responsible Medicine calculates that 63 percent of taxpayer farm subsidies directly benefit animal food producers.

Meanwhile, the small family farms who ostensibly are meant to be the primary recipients of aid are being left behind. Though taxpayers spent $161 billion in direct farm subsidies between 1995 and 2009, two-thirds of American farmers received nothing. Because the vast majority of subsidies go to the major corporations, who are then able to depress prices so significantly, a USDA study found that most small farms cannot sustain themselves.

How do fruit and vegetable farmers fare in all this? After all, as one study found, if all Americans were to follow the USDA healthy-eating guidelines, we would require an additional 13 million acres of fruit and vegetable crops. Yet farmers who grow fruits, vegetables, and nuts receive zero regular direct subsidies. Meanwhile, farmers who grow soybeans, corn, and other crops used for animal feed enjoy record paydays. In fact, many of these farmers don't grow *any* crops—they merely live on eligible land. (Even the billionaire media mogul Ted Turner receives a farm subsidy.) As the policy director for the National Sustainable Agriculture Coalition notes, "We've locked up food production with a policy that says, 'Thou shalt not grow fruits and vegetables.'"

DUBIOUS NUTRITION

We know the detrimental effects of animal products on our health thanks to independent, peer-reviewed studies.

The animal food industry knows the scientific studies as well. That's why they fund their own studies claiming that meat, eggs, fish, and dairy are good for you. Dr. Michael Greger analyzes nutrition studies and separates the science from the pseudoscience. He loves to point out a seemingly legitimate study published in the *American Journal of Clinical Nutrition,* "Beef in an Optimal Lean Diet [BOLD] Study: Effects on Lipids, Lipoproteins, and Apolipoproteins," which tries to prove that beef can reduce heart disease risk by lowering cholesterol. But as Dr. Greger explains, this study was "bought and paid for by the beef industry." The authors are forced to use incredibly dubious methods to arrive at this conclusion: While it is true that study participants did eat slightly more beef, they also removed most poultry, pork, fish, and cheese from their diet. So even with the added beef, participants reduced their overall animal protein and net saturated fat intake significantly—for saturated fat, they cut consumption in half—not your normal outcome for your average person who increases her beef intake! In short, they added more beef but cut out all the rest of the animal stuff, and all that other animal stuff is loaded with cholesterol and saturated fat. So guess what the study showed?

Unsurprisingly, participants' cholesterol levels improved, because saturated fat is a leading cause of high cholesterol, and saturated fat levels dropped with the overall drop in meat consumption. This allowed the researchers to assert, "The results of the BOLD study provide convincing evidence that lean beef can be included in a heart-healthy diet that meets current dietary recommendations and reduces cardiovascular disease risk." As Dr. Greger jokes, the beef could have been substituted for Crisco or Krispy Kreme donuts, and their cholesterol levels still would have dropped.

You see this all the time. Another study published in the *American Journal of Clinical Nutrition* starts promisingly enough: "Cheese intake in large amounts lowers LDL-cholesterol concentrations." Just don't read the second half of that title: "Compared with Butter Intake of Equal Fat Content." As Dr. Greger writes, "That's like touting the health benefits of Coca-Cola because it has less sugar than Pepsi."

THE REAL HEALTH COSTS, EXPOSED

We're only scratching the surface of how burdensome the standard American diet is not just to our health but to our economy. For a full picture, consider what are known as "externalized" costs. Let's say you buy a pack of cigarettes that costs you $8. The Centers for Disease Control and Prevention calculate that each pack carries with it a hidden charge of $10.47, paid for by American society at large—that's the economic impact of everything from lung infections to cancer treatment to countless other chronic diseases that require medical care. Taxpayers and people paying health insurance premiums pick up the tab.

By the same token, we're also picking up the tab for the externalized costs associated with eating animal-based protein—estimated at $414 billion annually. That means every $1 you spend on meat, dairy, fish, and eggs represents a $1.70 charge for everyone else. Maybe you've read this book and decided to pivot to clean protein. That's fantastic—but you'll still be paying the health costs for your neighbor who regularly opts for the surf and turf. If a member of Congress suggested that American taxpayers help fund cigarette advertisements or subsidize cigarettes for sale to schoolchildren, there would be an uproar. But that is exactly what we do for animal food companies.

Is Meat the New Tobacco?

The animal food industry has torn out dozens of pages from the Big Tobacco playbook. From denying scientific research to lobbying lawmakers to influencing health-care professionals, the industry is emulating the means by which tobacco companies convinced Americans that smoking was healthy—even long after the science declared otherwise. Let's review some of the parallels.

Step one in the playbook is denial. In 1964, the surgeon general declared that cigarette smoking caused lung cancer. The tobacco industry settled on a single counterattack: "Doubt is our product." Tobacco companies spent enormous amounts of money launching marketing campaigns to deny the cigarette-cancer link. From misleading "educational" films to flamboyantly untruthful advertising, the tobacco industry managed to discredit the science to keep Americans

continues

Is Meat the New Tobacco? *continued*

hooked on their product. As late as 1994, tobacco executives claimed under oath to Congress that "nicotine is not addictive." The meat industry is taking much the same tack today. In 2015 the World Health Organization condemned processed meat as a group-one human carcinogen—a class that includes tobacco products—and further concluded that red meat was probably carcinogenic. The North American Meat Institute immediately decried the WHO's findings as a "dramatic and alarmist overreach." The National Cattlemen's Beef Association trotted out its "experts," who complained that the WHO report was based on "weak associations" to the association's own nutritionist, who declared, "As a registered dietitian and mother, my advice hasn't changed."

Step two from the tobacco playbook is distortion. After the surgeon general's 1964 report, tobacco companies established the Tobacco Industry Research Committee among other shell organizations designed to manipulate the science. "Correlation is not causation" became the rallying cry. They blamed car exhaust and pollution for the increase in lung cancer deaths. Even as late as 1988, the CEO of Philip Morris claimed that the tobacco-cancer link was "only a statistical association. It has never been proven." As we've seen in this chapter, the meat industry either twists the data or funds its own studies that conveniently find no problem with meat consumption. After the WHO report, the National Cattlemen's Beef Association issued a press release with the petulant headline: "Science Does Not Support International Agency Opinion on Red Meat and Cancer." It cited a study conducted on behalf of the Beef Checkoff that concluded that "red meat does not appear to be an independent predictor" of cancer risk. The industry pointed to studies that show meat is safe, largely ignoring the weight of the science supporting the WHO findings.

continues

Is Meat the New Tobacco? *continued*

Step three is to throw all semblance of shame out the window. At times, the tobacco industry claimed that smoking was actually healthy. There were the infamous "More doctors smoke Camels than any other cigarette" advertisements. Lucky Strike declared that "20,679 physicians say 'Luckies are less irritating'" because they "protect the throat against cough." Philip Morris even ran ads declaring, "An ounce of prevention is worth a pound of cure: Philip Morris cigarettes are scientifically proved far less irritating to the nose and throat." Likewise, the meat industry claims that animal products are "high-quality protein" and "rich in nutrients." They even assert that "processed meats offer good nutrition."

As Stanford science historian Dr. Robert N. Proctor writes in the *New York Times*, with respect to climate change deniers, "We now live in a world where ignorance of a very dangerous sort is being deliberately manufactured, to protect certain kinds of unfettered corporate enterprise." Tobacco companies deliberately distorted science to preserve their profit margins, just like animal food companies distort nutrition science to preserve theirs. During the early 1990s, a US district judge overseeing a tobacco industry case declared, "All too often in the choice between the physical health of consumers and the financial well-being of business, concealment is chosen over disclosure, sales over safety, and money over morality."

RESET: A REFRESHED GOAL

Even when you don't see eye-to-eye with people who work in the animal food industry, you can talk heart-to-heart with them. Those industries are made up of people who are in all important ways just like you; they want to do good and live with purpose while at the same time provide a life for their families.

We have met many people who work in the meat industry, and we can say with conviction that the people who work in the meat industry genuinely believe they are helping the world. The Green Revolution during the mid-twentieth century developed fertilizers and pesticides that vastly improved global food production. "Feed the world" became the entire agricultural industry's mantra. Putting food on tables in America and around the world is noble work. Today's globalized animal food corporations were born from that well-meaning idea, and that good intent remains. With the proliferation of clean protein, there is a way for them—from small farmers to the CEOs of big corporations—to invest and adapt for the next iteration of "feeding the world."

We want to be really clear, here: It is easy to vilify the animal food industry as some sort of monolithic force intent on destroying our health and our environment. That is not true. Mom-and-pop dairy farmers in Vermont are not to blame for our current health crisis, and neither are executives working for the meat industry. And as we will discuss in Chapters 10 and 11, the meat industry will be essential to any plan that will successfully flip our national and global consumption patterns. Basically, we envision a meat industry that focuses on plant-based and "clean meat," but more on both of those market sectors in Chapters 9 and 10.

PART 2
The Clean Protein Solution

CHAPTER 5

The Lean, Mean Bean

The cornerstone of every longevity diet in the world
is quite simply: beans.
—Dan Buettner, National Geographic
fellow and founder of the Blue Zones

In 2004, longevity researcher Dan Buettner began studying the
regions of the world with the healthiest and happiest people.
Eventually he identified five "Blue Zones" populations that enjoy especially long and healthy lives. Dan went on to write three
New York Times best sellers about the nine key characteristics of
the longest-lived and happiest people in the world; we recommend
them highly. The zones differ modestly in terms of diet, but two
factors remain constant: all of these populations consumed 90 percent or greater whole plant foods, and they ate at least a cup of
beans every single day.

As just one example of a bean believer, ever since President Bill
Clinton adopted a predominantly plant-based diet in 2010, he
has been all about beans, as he explained to Wolf Blitzer during a
CNN interview: "I live on beans, legumes, vegetables, [and] fruit."

The former president adopted his mostly plant-based diet—he still eats a bit of fish every few weeks or so—after reading *The China Study* by T. Colin Campbell and *Prevent and Reverse Heart Disease* by Dr. Caldwell Esselstyn. He received nutritional counseling from Dr. Dean Ornish.

As Clinton explained to Blitzer, going plant based "changed my whole metabolism and I lost 24 pounds. I got back to basically what I weighed in high school. . . . I did all this research, and I saw that 82 percent of the people since 1986 who have gone on a plant-based diet, no dairy, no meat, of any kind, no chicken, no turkey, have begun to heal themselves." Clinton's weight loss was typical: a study of the only Blue Zone in the United States, the Adventists of Loma Linda, California, found that this plant-based population weighed an average of 30 pounds less than those who included meat in their diet. Similarly, there was a linear relationship between animal product consumption and diabetes.

PROTEIN

Beans have been staples around the world for most of human history, not only because they're cheap, versatile, and delicious, but also because they're high in protein, fiber, iron, and antioxidants. They fill you up, make you feel strong and energetic, and keep you healthy. Not that the folks in ancient cultures thought much about it, but beans happen to be low on the glycemic index, are gluten-free, and have been associated with lower cholesterol, balanced blood sugar, and digestive regularity. In Latin America you'll see black beans served with corn, while in the Middle East you'll regularly enjoy hummus with bread, and all over Asia there's plenty of tofu and soy products mixed into the daily fare.

Beans are absolutely packed with protein, but they don't have all the saturated fat, cholesterol, toxins, and other harmful ingredients in animal products that piggyback on protein. Some will point out that plant protein is attached to fiber, which inhibits some absorption. This is actually true—if you're getting your protein from beans rather than animals, you'll need a bit more of it. But, as we already discussed, if you are eating a normal amount of calories, you are already receiving plenty of protein. Remember, *almost all whole foods have protein!*

For you diehards out there, one option to maximize your protein intake is to break down the fibrous cells walls by soaking or sprouting the beans. For those of you who are numbers minded, soaking whole peas for six hours increases protein availability by 8 percent. If you soak them for eighteen hours and then put them through a pressure cooker, the protein will be 33 percent more bioavailable. But if you're like us, sprouting is just way too much trouble. You still get all the protein you need from good old canned beans!

COMPLEX CARBS AND FIBER

Beans also have something critical that meat does not: complex carbohydrates and fiber. Simple carbohydrates are just what they sound like: carbohydrates with a simple chemical structure of just one or two sugars, often referred to as monosaccharides and disaccharides. You often find simple carbohydrates in soda, energy drinks, syrup, and candy. If you are athletic, it is fine to obtain some portion of your calories from simple sugars, but, generally, simple sugars crowd out foods that have useful nutrients and should be avoided.

The most important nutrients, which should make up the bulk of your caloric intake, are complex carbohydrates. They are called "complex" because they have three or more linked sugars, referred to as oligosaccharides and polysaccharides. Whole foods with plenty of complex carbohydrates, such as legumes, are the healthiest; they are almost always packed with fiber, vitamins, minerals, and phytochemicals.

Fiber is also critical, and most Americans are not getting nearly enough of it. Fiber is the part of plant food that is not digested; rather, it passes through and cleans you out. There's an old wives' tale about meat sitting in your colon for years, and although it's not true, it stems from the fact that meat has no fiber, so people who eat a lot of meat and very few plants can go days without a bowel movement.

There are two types of fiber: soluble and insoluble. Both are plentiful in plant-based foods, especially beans. Soluble fiber dissolves in water—hence the name—and helps with cholesterol levels, blood pressure, and glucose levels. Insoluble fiber does not change form in your digestive tract; it moves through intact and helps clean the lining of your intestines and promote regular bowel movements. Fiber can also help you avoid developing minor health problems such as hemorrhoids or constipation, while helping to prevent major disease including colon cancer and heart disease. One study published in the journal *Stroke* finds that increasing your fiber intake by 7 grams a day—the equivalent of a ½ cup serving of baked beans—can lower your risk of stroke by 7 percent. In another study, Yale University researchers find that premenopausal women who ate 6 or more grams of soluble fiber daily (just a cup of black beans) had 62 percent lower odds of breast cancer compared with women who ate less than 4 grams.

The Academy of Nutrition and Dietetics recommends 25 grams of fiber per day for women and 38 grams for men. If you are consuming at least five servings of fruit and vegetables every day and basing your entrées around whole foods, you should easily meet that recommendation. However, as we've discussed, the standard American diet includes very few beans, grains, and vegetables, and quite a lot of meat, eggs, and dairy—none of which has any fiber whatsoever. Please allow us to underline that point: meat, dairy, and eggs have no fiber at all.

That may explain why the average American consumes only 15 grams of fiber per day, which is 60 percent of the recommendation for women and well under half of the recommendation for men. "Where do you get your protein?" may be a common question for someone who is cutting back on their meat intake, but no one ever asks a heavy meat-eater "Where do you get your fiber?" even though a fiber-deficient diet has been linked to heart disease, cancer, diabetes, obesity, and other chronic diseases endemic in Western countries—and even though most Americans already get too little of this vital nutrient.

Note that in addition to being super protein sources, beans are also great sources of fiber. For example, just half a cup of cooked black beans contains 7.5 grams of fiber. Kidney beans, lima beans, navy beans, pinto beans, and lentils contain even more. If you are also eating five servings of fruits and vegetables—as everyone should—and a handful of nuts every day (more in the next chapter), you should be taking in all the fiber you need.

BEANS DECREASE YOUR RISK OF CHRONIC DISEASE

Beans are a great source of vitamins and minerals. Of course, we all know that vitamins and minerals are essential to health: they build strong bones, allow us to heal after we get injured, and ensure that we have a functioning immune system. Considering the exemplary nutritional profile of beans, it's not surprising that the studies find that they decrease your risk of heart disease, cancer, diabetes, and obesity.

Commenting on the fact that beans are considered to be both a legume and a vegetable by the USDA, Dr. Greger, author of the indispensable book *How Not to Die*, writes, "You get the best of both worlds with beans, all the while enjoying foods that are naturally low in saturated fat and sodium and free of cholesterol." And the Academy of Nutrition and Dietetics adds, "Beans and lentils not only provide protein but are an excellent source of fiber, vitamins and minerals, while being low in fat and having no cholesterol. Buy them dried, canned, frozen or fresh."

The biggest killer in the West is heart disease, and many studies have shown that legume consumption can lower your risk. For example, one study in the *Journal of Nutrition* finds that just a ⅓ cup serving of beans per day lowered the heart attack risk by 38 percent among 2,000 study participants who had already suffered cardiac episodes. Another study, this one published in the *Archives of Internal Medicine*, determines that participants who ate four servings of beans per week lowered their heart disease risk by 22 percent over those who ate none among a group of almost 10,000 men and women who had no signs of heart disease at the outset of the study.

The number two killer in the West is cancer, the incidence of which is also consistently found to be inversely proportional to bean consumption and positively associated with meat consumption. For example, research published in the journal *Cancer Research* reviewed epidemiological work on cancer across forty-one countries and finds "strong and consistent correlations . . . between death rates of cancers of the colon and breast and the per capita consumption of total fat and of nutrients derived from animal sources." The same study finds that bean consumption was linked to lower rates of colon, breast, and prostate cancer. In 2007, the American Institute for Cancer Research published the results of a comprehensive look at every study of diet and cancer ever done. Among their recommendations for prevention of cancer is the consumption of beans at every meal. As Dr. Greger puts it, "Not every day or every week. Every meal!"

WEIGHT LOSS

Trying to lose weight? Adding beans to your diet can help!

In one study conducted by scientists at Purdue and Bastyr Universities, with calories held steady, adding 3 cups of beans or lentils per week (about one serving per day) more than tripled average weight loss from 2 to more than 7 pounds. In another study from the *European Journal of Nutrition,* calorie-restricted diets that included four servings of beans per week were associated with 50 percent more weight loss than diets with the same level of restricted calories but no beans. Simply put: participants took in exactly the same number of calories, but the participants who were consuming beans lost a lot more weight.

Since people who consume beans have lower rates of obesity and other chronic diseases, it only makes sense that they would live longer. Sure enough, the title of a study in the *Asia Pacific Journal of Clinical Nutrition* sums up the case: "Legumes: The Most Important Dietary Predictor of Survival in Older People of Different Ethnicities." The researchers looked at five cohorts in four countries over seven years and found that every 20 grams of increased daily legume consumption was associated with a decrease in 7–8 percent mortality. Twenty grams of beans is about ¼ cup, or slightly less than one serving per day. Of course, the American Institute of Cancer Research recommends three servings per day. Now we know why.

A FEW WORDS ABOUT GAS

"Beans, beans, good for your heart. . . . " Yes, we know that beans have a gassy reputation, but most people who add beans to their diets find that their systems acclimate, and they pass less gas over time. For example, researchers asked study participants to consume

Gas Busters

Gas happens. Everyone gets it, and it's natural. In fact, gas is a good sign that you're eating a proper amount of fiber. Don't worry if you're experiencing more gas than usual; your body will get used to the healthy legumes, vegetables, grains, and fruits. In the meantime, try any of the following:

1. **Take a daily probiotic supplement.** Many studies show that restoring the gut's good bacteria will significantly reduce gas and bloating. Also try probiotic-rich foods, like fresh fruits and vegetables.
2. **Pop a couple digestive enzymes with your meal.** They'll help break down your food and reduce the bloat.
3. **Add a few drops of bitters**—yes, the same ones you make cocktails with—to a bit of water and drink them before a meal. The bitterness will signal your digestive system to go to work. Gastric juices will gear up for action and stimulate the release of your own body's digestive enzymes.
4. **Whole fruit is fine, but steer clear of added sugars**— they promote bacterial overgrowth and gas.
5. **Soak your beans overnight and switch out the water before cooking them slowly and for a long time.** Make sure they're soft and not crunchy before eating. Add a few pieces of kombu while cooking, too, as the amino acids in the sea vegetable help break down the heavy starches in the beans, helping them move through your body more easily.

½ cup of beans daily for eight or twelve weeks—a bit more than one serving per day. The study was focused on heart disease, but participants also filled out a weekly questionnaire that included analysis of flatulence, stool changes, and bloating. Throughout the various trials, fewer than half of the participants reported increased gas in the first week, and, of those who did, 70 percent reported that the gas went away within two to three weeks.

That said, if you're eating beans and experiencing gas, there are a variety of things you can do. The first, as already implied, is to eat more of them: as your body becomes more accustomed to consuming legumes, it will get better at processing them. Additionally, soaking and rinsing beans and cooking them thoroughly will make them less likely to cause gas. Finally, many people have found that cooking beans with seaweed, especially kombu, will remove the substances that cause gas. Food writer for the *Washington Post* Casey Seidenberg explains that seaweed "contains enzymes that help break down the raffinose sugars in beans, which are the gas-producing culprits. Once they are broken down, we are able to absorb more of the nutrients, and we can enjoy these legumes without as many intestinal complaints."

CHAPTER 6

Nuts:
Power Packs of Nutrition

I love nuts, I'm for nuts, I am nuts.
—PENN JILLETTE

Okay, the talking half of Penn and Teller was actually refer-
ring to nutty people with nutty ideas who all seem to seek
him out for advice about said ideas, but we are—in fact—nuts for
nuts, which are a superb source of clean protein. And Mr. Jillette
is, too. Let's take a step back and note that the notoriously antiani-
mal comedian once did an entire TV program devoted to mocking
veganism and vegans as extreme killjoys. The only benefit of veganism was to one's health, but, for Jillette, that was definitely not
enough to make up for the lack of humor and heavy judgment that
he thought characterized vegetarians and vegans.

The health bit on the show was pretty funny. Jillette would es-
sentially say, "Look at me—fat, pale, and unhealthy—*obviously*
not plant-based!" And then the camera would flash to vegans such
as Ryan Gosling and Natalie Portman, nodding to the idea that

eating plants leads to attractiveness and energy, whereas eating a lot of meat is likely to make you fat and lethargic. It was funny but also quite sad. Jillette was basically arguing that you couldn't be healthy and sociable at the same time.

Now, with the help of his plant-based nutrition coach, Jillette knows better. He realized a few years back that clocking in at more than 330 pounds was a sure ticket to heart failure, and so he went on a plant-based and calorie-restricted diet, which allowed him to get down to a healthy weight. By sticking with a reasonable plant-based diet, Jillette writes, "I get focused and clearer and . . . well, happier." The funny man and magic iconoclast has kept the weight off by focusing on plant foods, especially nuts, which he says keep him feeling full. When he eats nuts, he won't crave the saturated fat–filled foods that he used to eat.

In case you're wondering, Jillette's nuts of choice are peanuts (stickler alert: technically a legume!), peanut butter (legume butter!), flax, and chia seeds. And indeed, Jillette was onto something. Nuts are a bit of a miracle food. They are, as you almost certainly know, very high in protein. Peanuts, flaxseeds, and sesame seeds are 17 percent protein, and almonds and pistachios are 15 percent protein. Soy nuts are a whopping 40 percent protein. There is almost as much protein in just 1 ounce of most nuts and seeds as an entire cup of skim milk.

However, unlike animal-based protein sources, nuts are also packed with complex carbohydrates and fiber. (To repeat, animal foods have a grand total of zero complex carbohydrates and zero fiber.) If your goal is to maintain a healthy weight with plenty of energy while decreasing your likelihood of contracting heart disease, cancer, or diabetes, you want to be eating plenty of complex carbohydrates and plenty of fiber.

Nuts are also rich in healthy polyunsaturated and monounsaturated fats. Though unfairly maligned, nonsaturated fats are critical for a functioning metabolism, help supply energy, help us absorb critical vitamins and minerals, and are critical components of our cell membranes. Fat gets a bad rap because of *saturated* and *trans* fat, which are linked to heart disease, diabetes, obesity, and many other ailments. There is no nutritional requirement for any saturated or trans fat, and most nutritional bodies recommend that consumers eat no more than 10 percent of their calories in saturated fat. Many recommend zero.

Meat and dairy tend to be high in saturated fats, with dairy fat mostly clocking in at over 60 percent saturated. Chicken fat is just over one-third saturated, which is a bit more than beef and a bit less than pork. Fish is sometimes touted for its low saturated fat levels compared to other animal products, but fish fat is still 20 percent or more saturated.

HEART DISEASE

Because of their healthy fats, nuts are extremely good for your heart. Nuts tend to be high in unsaturated fats, omega-3 fats, and fiber, all three of which lower LDL cholesterol and reduce arterial inflammation—both of which are linked to arterial clogging. Omega-3 fatty acids also appear to prevent abnormal heart rhythms that can lead to sudden cardiac death.

A study published in 2016 in the prestigious journal *JAMA Internal Medicine* reviewed the link between diet and disease for more than 80,000 women and 40,000 men, all health professionals, and confirmed that eating high amounts of saturated fat increases the likelihood of premature death. The study found that replacing saturated fat with unsaturated fat, such as those found in nuts, can decrease mortality by 27 percent. That is really quite remarkable—imagine if the nut industry had the lobbying power in Washington of the meat industry!

Nuts also contain heavy doses of plant sterols and L-arginine, both of which improve blood flow and make your arterial walls more supple, decreasing the risk of heart disease, stroke, and other blood-flow related diseases. A 2014 meta-analysis in the *British Journal of Nutrition* reviewed more than 120 studies and determined that small amounts of plant sterols can lower LDL cholesterol by an average of 12 percent.

WEIGHT LOSS

Nuts contain a variety of nutrients that make them a great source of fat and calories for everyone, but especially for athletes and people who are trying to lose weight. When Bruce first adopted a plant-based diet in 1987, he was playing a lot of sports and running cross-country. He weighed 175 pounds, and Big Macs from McDonald's and Blizzards from DQ were a significant part of his daily fare. When he stopped eating high-calorie meat and dairy products, he quickly dropped to about 165 pounds. While he felt great and had even more energy, his friends joked that he had some sort of disease. Enter the remarkable superfood: the nut. Since 1987, Bruce has been consuming about a cup of nuts per day, and, in addition to all the long-term benefits, nuts allow him to take in enough calories on a daily basis to sustain his active lifestyle. Unlike meat and dairy, nuts can be eaten just before a workout or a long bike ride. Kathy is also a big fan of nuts, heaping a huge spoonful of nut butter into her daily smoothies, having an apple with peanut butter almost every afternoon, and snacking on nuts that are always tucked away in her car and handbag. She, too, was considerably heavier when her diet focused on animal foods but lost the weight and kept it off without effort after shifting to nonanimal foods.

Counterintuitively, nuts are also great for weight loss. Indeed, Penn Jillette's weight loss experience has been backed up by scientific studies. For example, a 2010 review found that adding nuts to your diet helps with both weight loss and weight maintenance. The authors speculated that even though nuts are calorically dense and high in fat, their fiber content increases satiety. Nuts were also found to increase resting metabolism, meaning your body will naturally burn more calories when at rest.

Jillette also mentions feeling mentally more clear when he had eaten nuts, in large part because they allowed him to feel full without feeling stuffed. Indeed, nuts tend to be very high in vitamin E and the B vitamin folate, which helps to prevent deterioration of cognitive function. Interestingly, one of the better nuts for this effect is peanuts, which is Jillette's favorite. Even more interesting, the *British Journal of Nutrition* finds a link between walnut consumption and immediately improved working memory, which includes the ability to solve problems, and motor function.

In 2016, researchers from Imperial College London and the Norwegian University of Science and Technology pored over twenty-nine studies involving 819,000 participants, concluding in peer-reviewed research published in *BMC Medicine* that "people who eat at least 20 grams of nuts a day have a lower risk of heart disease, cancer and other diseases." That's ¼ cup of nuts, which could easily be tossed onto a salad or into your morning smoothie if you have a Vitamix (more in Chapter 9). That mere ¼ cup of nuts cut heart disease risk by 30 percent, cancer risk by 15 percent, and risk of premature death by 22 percent. Nut intake "was also associated with a reduced risk of dying from respiratory disease by about a half, and diabetes by nearly 40 percent."

Specific nuts have been found to have specific benefits, though we suspect that a study indicating that one nut has a certain benefit is likely to apply to other nuts. It's hard to know for certain just which nutrient in a whole food is responsible for an observed effect, and we agree with Michael Pollan and Mark Bittman that, most likely, the beneficial effects of one food are the beneficial effects of *food*—not of specific nutrients that can be isolated and turned into pills and shots.

And that analysis only makes the scientific work with specific nuts all the more interesting. For example, pistachios have been linked to a lower risk of lung cancer, perhaps due to high levels of vitamin E (many nuts have high levels of the vitamin) and Brazil nuts to a lower risk for prostate cancer, perhaps due to high levels of selenium. Walnuts appear to improve the "vitality, motility, and morphology" of sperm, and pistachios appear to reduce erectile dysfunction. If you monitor the health pages of your local paper, you'll see studies along these lines on a fairly constant basis. But what you won't see is any study indicating health harms from nut consumption, absent allergies.

All these benefits from nuts add up to something unsurprising—a lower risk of mortality and chronic disease generally, according to a study in the *International Journal of Epidemiology*. The study included 120,000 men and women over a period of almost twenty years, and finds that daily consumption of nuts—including peanuts— was linked to "substantially lower mortality" at a consumption of 15 grams per day or more. The key benefits from nut consumption are reduced risk from "respiratory disease, neurodegenerative disease, and diabetes, followed by cancer and cardiovascular diseases."

The takeaway: Eat nuts, and enjoy them. Eat almonds and cashews and walnuts and pistachios and any other nut you can get your hands on. And, assuming that our good friend Penn Jillette keeps up the nut consumption, we are going to have him around for quite some time to laugh with.

CHAPTER 7

Diversify

There's no need to plan meals around complementary proteins. In 2009, the Academy of Nutrition and Dietetics (AND) released a paper stating that eating a variety of plant foods over the course of the day provides all the required amino acids. The Centers for Disease Control and Prevention agrees with AND and discredits the rumor that humans need to eat certain proteins together to receive adequate nutrition.

—Physicians Committee for
Responsible Medicine (PCRM)

In 1971, Frances Moore Lappé published her groundbreaking book *Diet for a Small Planet*, which argued that cycling grains through animals so that humans can eat those animals is a vastly inefficient method of producing protein. She asserted that the system was wasteful, that it contributed to global poverty, and that readers could change the world by changing their diets. She was the first to make the argument in a way that resonated with the public, but she was certainly not the last.

Another argument that Lappé made in her book has had equal staying power, though she later renounced it: that plant protein must be complemented in order to be made "whole" and accessible to the same degree as animal-based proteins. In short, the idea is that some foods—say, legumes—have an amino acid profile that is incomplete and must be made complete by adding complementary plant-based proteins at the same meal—say, from whole grains.

The notion that we need to complement proteins does not, however, have any scientific backing at all. As discussed in Chapter 2, we have no need to consume animal proteins, and there is no one in a developed country who is suffering from protein deficiency, no matter what they eat. Considering that there are millions of vegans in the United States alone, if protein complementing were necessary, there would be some scientific evidence by now. But there is none.

So it is remarkable how often nutritionists and dietitians continue to perpetuate the myth that plant-based proteins must be combined to satisfy protein needs. You would think they must see patients who are suffering from inadequate protein intake, and yet they don't see such patients ever, because these people do not exist, unless they are also suffering from malnutrition based in inadequate caloric consumption. The diseases that plague us are not diseases of deficiency; they are diseases of overconsumption, like heart disease, cancer, and obesity. How many people have you ever met who are protein deficient while eating enough food? None. How many people have you met who are overweight or obese? If you're like most Americans, plenty.

TO COMBINE OR NOT TO COMBINE?

The idea of complementing protein does make some intuitive sense, which may account for its staying power: There are twenty amino acids that make up protein, and nine "essential" amino acids must come from food. Animal products are so-called complete proteins because they have lots of all nine amino acids you are supposed to consume. Some plants are complete too, including soy, buckwheat, and quinoa.

Most grains are low in lysine, and most legumes are low in tryptophan, methionine, and cysteine. Fortunately, legumes are high in lysine, and grains are high in tryptophan, methionine, and cysteine. So as long as you eat some grains and some legumes, you'll get some of each essential amino acid. The difference is that Lappé originally thought this was required at every meal. In fact, as long you don't eat *only* grains or *only* beans, you will perfectly fine!

A similarly unnecessary food consumption technique involves combining foods not with a focus on protein but on general health, digestion, energy, and other reasons. We should take a step back and note that although we have met many people who are devotees of plans focusing on food combining—for instance, only eating fruit in the morning and twenty minutes before any other food, or eating nuts and dried fruit with raw vegetables—combining certain foods for best digestion or maximum protein absorption appears unnecessary, according to the best science. If you do a Google search for "food combining," you will find, like much on the Internet, completely contradictory information. For example, "10 Common Food Combinations That Wreak Havoc on Your Health" and "Food Combining Diet Is a Myth: Don't Be Fooled" are back to back at numbers two and three. Of course, what neither of these sites offers is a citation to even a single journal article that would corroborate its faith in food combining.

While it may be true that some people feel better when they adopt food combining principles, that's almost certainly because these programs also recommend eating whole foods. For example, Fit for Life is a completely plant-based program. So, sure, if you go from the standard American diet to a diet based on whole plant foods, you're likely to feel better with or without food combining.

In what may be the only study done on food combining, from the *International Journal of Obesity* in 2000, two sets of subjects were placed on the same nutritionally adequate but calorically restricted diet, one set following food combining principles and the other not. The subjects who combined their foods according to the principles lost slightly less weight, but the numbers were not statistically significant. The study's authors concluded what science has been telling us consistently: *what* you eat is important, not the order in which you eat it.

PERFECT PROTEIN MEALS
YOU MAY ALREADY BE ENJOYING

You really don't need to think about combining foods in order to get the perfect protein. If you eat healthy, plant-based foods over the course of the day or even week, you'll get what you need. Just to show you how *not* difficult this is, here are a few nuggets of perfection you might already have in your kitchen rotation:

- Oatmeal topped with nuts or seeds
- Acai bowl topped with granola/oats, seeds, and nuts
- Salad with hemp seeds
- Granola (oats, nuts, dried fruits)
- Burritos (whole wheat wrap with black beans, rice, and vegetables)
- Veg tacos (whole wheat flour or corn tortilla, beans or tofu scramble or plant-based meat crumble with veggies and salsa)
- Red lentil soup (red lentils, barley, parsley)
- Curry (vegetables, tofu, rice)

- Sushi (rice and vegetables and tofu)
- Cereal (sprouted grains and seeds, nuts)
- Sprouted bread topped with almond butter and sliced banana
- Zucchini and noodles topped with green lentils
- Plant-based or bean burger on whole wheat bun with a side salad
- Quinoa with wild mushrooms and broccoli (note: quinoa, buckwheat, and soy are already complete proteins)
- Carrots, celery, and peppers with hummus or baba ghanoush and pita bread
- Chili (beans, vegetables, and rice)
- Tabouleh (vegetables and bulgur) with fava or garbanzo beans
- Dolma/sarma (vegetables—peppers, tomatoes, zucchini—stuffed with rice and kidney beans)
- Beet/carrot shredded salad with quinoa, sunflower seeds, cashew nuts
- Veggie stir-fry with tofu and noodles
- Polenta with tempeh and eggplant sprinkled with olive oil
- Couscous, tofu, and vegetables with balsamic vinaigrette
- Panini with hummus, eggplant, tomatoes, and olive oil
- Falafel with pita bread, hummus, and side salad

WHAT ABOUT TIMING YOUR FOOD CONSUMPTION?

If you read the muscle mags, you might think that you have to precisely time your protein intake to maximize fat burning and muscle gain. Is choosing when and how you eat your protein the difference between being a flabby weakling and a muscle-bound bodybuilder? Some science indicates that protein before a workout is ideal, and some suggests postworkout. Many bodybuilding columns take a very firm stance on one or the other, but if they cite studies at all, they do so very selectively. The one thing that's absolutely true is that if you're an athlete, you need more calories, and so you need more protein. How and when you ingest it will probably have little effect on your muscles and recovery time.

An analysis in the journal *Nutrition Research Review* finds that students who consume breakfast generally have better nutrient intakes and maintain healthier weights, and that adding breakfast to nonbreakfast regimes tends to improve cognition and academic performance. But the study does not clearly indicate that the time of consumption was responsible for the positive results. Indeed, a review of forty-five peer-reviewed studies found that positive results for breakfast consumption are largely due to increased nutrient levels overall, not timing; the effect in students who were already consuming adequate nutrition was negligible. Similarly, breakfast's positive academic outcome may be a result of the program getting kids to school in the first place.

The takeaway is eat healthy, clean protein when you are hungry. Don't worry about when the *when* or the *how*.

DIVERSIFY

If you look around the world, complementing proteins does appear to be a natural way of eating. In Latin America, you will find people pairing beans with tortillas. In the Middle East you'll see pita and hummus, bulgur and chickpeas. Throughout much of Asia you will find soy and rice, and in India, lentils with rice or bread. And all across the good ole United States, you'll find peanut butter on bread—one of our favorite complete proteins. But these truths mask a larger truth: it is very, very hard to be protein deficient if you consume enough calories to sustain yourself. As

Frances Moore Lappé declares in the tenth anniversary edition of her book, "If people are getting enough calories, they are virtually certain of getting enough protein."

As cookbook author and food guru Mark Bittman is fond of saying, "Don't eat lycopene; eat a tomato. Don't eat protein; eat a bean burrito." When we try to isolate the precise nutritional benefit of certain foods, sometimes we may be right, but often we will be wrong. That's why supplements, which extract ingredients with purported health benefits from whole foods, often don't work. For example, turmeric is a famed spice that has been linked to reduced cancer risk, and many researchers believe its active ingredient, curcumin, is the reason. But supplements containing only curcumin have been less successful, meaning there is more to the magic of turmeric than we understand.

That's why it's so important to consume whole foods. For instance, we've known for decades that oats protect against heart disease, but we don't know whether it's the fiber, the magnesium, the folic acid, the phytochemicals, or how it all works in concert. Probably, oats are just one of nature's many perfect foods—especially if you add some mixed nuts on top.

Oats are just one example of whole-grain superfoods. Studies in the Western world also show a correlation between whole-grain consumption and reduced risk for heart disease, cancer, diabetes, and premature mortality. For example, in 2016, scientists from Harvard's School of Public Health and other top universities published a metareview in the *BMJ* of more than sixty publications; their conclusion is that just three servings of whole grains per day, which is the equivalent of three pieces of bread or 1.5 cups of oatmeal, "is associated with a reduced risk of coronary heart disease, cardiovascular disease, and total cancer, and mortality from all causes, respiratory diseases, infectious diseases, diabetes, and all non-cardiovascular, non-cancer causes."

While protein complementing is not necessary, one form of combining that does work is "food synergy" for maximum nutrient load. For example, you need fat in your diet to help you absorb fat-soluble vitamins, while vitamin C helps you absorb iron. One of the more interesting results about these foods working together is that carotenoid absorption in salads is enhanced by fat consumption. Carotenoids are the brightly colored pigments you see in fruits and vegetables, and they are linked to healthy skin, clear vision, cardiovascular health, and other health benefits. They are also packed with antioxidants, which fight off carcinogenic activity. A little can go a long way: a study out of Ohio State University and published in the *Journal of Nutrition* found that the addition of just 2.5 tablespoons of avocado to a carrot and spinach salad increased alpha-carotene absorption by more than 800 percent, beta-carotene absorption by 1,300 percent, and lutein absorption by more than 400 percent.

Consider this: twenty years ago, other than beta-carotene, scientists barely knew what a phytonutrient was. We hadn't discovered lycopene, which gives tomatoes much of their nutritional power, and we didn't know about pterostilbene, responsible (we think) for the nutritional power of blueberries. Indeed, researchers discover new information about the more than 100,000 phytonutrients in plants on a daily basis. Since we barely know what they are and what they do, it won't surprise you to learn that we also don't know about how these nutrients work together in food. Overall, what we know is that they work synergistically as a whole. You need not be a chemist!

If you're looking to pack some protein in your meal, don't discount brightly colored fruits. Most berries and citrus fruits hover at about 10 percent protein, and most vegetables pack quite a lot more. For example, kale and cauliflower are both low in protein by vegetable standards, but per calorie they still clock in at about

33 percent protein. Broccoli, spinach, zucchini, and mushrooms—and nearly all leafy greens and yellow vegetables—are 50 percent or more protein. Remember that vegetables are low in calories; you have to eat many of them to fulfill your daily caloric (and protein) needs. For best results, put them on a bed of brown rice or quinoa.

The Harvard T. H. Chan School of Public Health points out that a diet heavy in fruit and vegetables is linked with lower rates of heart disease, stroke, cancer, cataracts, digestive problems, and more. And, according to scientists writing in the *Journal of Nutrition*, more than 96 percent of Americans do not consume the USDA-recommended amount of legumes, whole grains, dark green vegetables, or orange vegetables. Summing up, the authors report that "dark green vegetables, orange vegetables, legumes, and whole grains had the poorest showing, with nearly everyone in each sex-age group failing to meet recommendations."

Considering that everybody gets enough protein and almost no one gets enough beans, whole grains, or leafy greens, the fact that we do not put more national focus on eating a wide variety of plant foods—"eating the rainbow"—is a flagrant example of what happens when you allow industry to control policy and education. You need not count calories, fat, protein grams or diligently look to combine certain amino acids, but instead eat from the plant-based rainbow spectrum of beans, nuts, vegetables, and whole grains. As long as you eat a normal amount of calories with a variety of plant foods, you will receive all the protein you need—not to mention a wealth of life-extending nutrients.

CHAPTER 8

Drink It

Recently, Kathy received an email from a close friend:

> I'm really struggling with eating healthily. . . . I feel like I'm cheating myself sometimes. Like, I'm hungry and I'm not sure I'm getting the nutrition I need. Not many great options where I live. I'm crazy busy with work, and I don't always have time to cook and prepare. . . . I need my protein. I'm working out hard. I want to feel grounded. Fed. Nourished.

Sound like anyone you know? After a few exchanges about how to deal with friends and restaurants, Kathy shared one of her secrets: "Here's my secret weapon, and I swear it keeps me so strong and nourished. I make a protein shake every day, so I never feel I haven't gotten my quota of nutrients."

After Kathy shared her recipe (see next page), her friend replied, "OMG that would cover protein, greens, omegas! You made my day; I'm so on it!"

Both of us spend a lot of time in airports and traveling to areas where healthy food is hard to find. One solution that we've found, in addition to the glories of Starbucks' oatmeal, is protein shakes and drinkable meals. Yes, we know, drinking your food leaves something to be desired. Very few people like food more than we do, and very few people are more committed to good food. However, we also live in the real world, and we don't want to spend ten dollars for ¼ cup of mixed nuts at the airport, and we don't always have time to cook.

Protein shakes and meals in a glass are a tidy solution in an imperfect world. Sometimes, eating in an ideal way is not possible, but there are some phenomenal plant-based protein powders and liquid meals that are healthy, affordable, and work in a pinch. They will also give you an energy boost as you rush out the door in the morning.

SMOOTHIES

We both enjoy a smoothie every day. As discussed in the previous chapter, breakfast consumption is not critical in itself, but for people who are not taking in enough calories or who are perpetually exhausted, adding a high-protein breakfast or postworkout snack can be incredibly helpful. We find that a nutrient-dense smoothie provides a nice boost of energy that lasts for hours.

Here is Bruce's favorite smoothie recipe for two: Place the following in a high speed blender: 2 pieces of whole fruit (e.g., 1 orange and 1 apple), 1 frozen banana, 1 cup of mixed berries, 2 cups of soy milk or Ripple (a plant-based milk), ½ cup of flaxseeds or walnuts. Blend for 60 seconds, and your smoothie is ready to be enjoyed. And yes, you want to put the whole flaxseeds in (as long as the blender is powerful; if not, use preground flaxseeds), the whole walnuts in, and all of that will blend to liquid.

Kathy's current obsession is this one, also for two people: coconut water, vanilla or berry plant-based protein powder (a full scoop of Vega Sport Performance), a heaping spoon of almond butter, a big handful each of frozen pineapple and strawberries, ground

flaxseeds, a couple handfuls of either frozen kale, spinach, or broccoli. Throw in some chia seeds, but just a small spoonful lest your
smoothie be too thick. Blend hard. Done.

Boom. You just met your entire day's USDA recommendation for fruit and omega-3 fatty acids, and most of your veggies.
You get 22 grams of plant-based protein from Bruce's recipe and
roughly 30 grams from Kathy's.

You might want to invest in a quality blender if you are consistently processing vegetables and nuts, which can do a number
on the more inexpensive blades. Both of us use Vitamix blenders, which are widely considered the best. Neither of us has stock
in Vitamix, but if the company were publicly traded, we certainly
would!

Don't Drink Sugar-in-a-Bottle Beverages

So, drinking smoothies is great. They're naturally sweet thanks
to the whole fruit, and thoroughly healthy. So does that mean
orange juice, Coca-Cola, apple juice, root beer, grape juice,
Gatorade, and other sweetened beverages are healthy? No!
This might come as a surprise. Is there really no difference
between Coca-Cola and apple juice?

Simple sugars are simple sugars, and some of the best aspects of fruit, like their mineral and fiber content, are eliminated when they are turned into juice. That is why research
consistently shows that although fruit consumption is associated with lower rates of obesity, diabetes, and chronic disease, fruit *juice* consumption goes in the other direction.

Think about this: a 16-ounce bottle of apple juice contains as many calories as a 20-ounce Coca-Cola and almost
as much sugar. And every flavored milk that we checked contains even more calories than Mountain Dew, plus no fiber,
no complex carbohydrates, and a lot of fat. Indeed, a study in
the journal *Appetite* shows that although fruit consumption

continues

Don't Drink Sugar-in-a-Bottle Beverages *continued*

lowers blood pressure, fruit juice consumption elevates it. The authors explain that "despite a common perception that fruit juice is healthy, fruit juice contains high amounts of naturally occurring sugar without the fibre content of the whole fruit." Similarly, a study published in the prestigious journal the *Lancet* points to a link between juice consumption and obesity that was identical to the link between soda consumption and obesity. The authors titled their analysis, "Fruit Juice: Just Another Sugary Drink?" The question is, of course, rhetorical.

Some of you eagle-eyed readers might be thinking, *Wait a minute, guys. How is fruit blended with a Vitamix healthy, while fruit juice you buy at the store is not healthy?* Good question! The answer is fiber and phytonutrients. When you blend a whole fruit, the fiber and phytonutrients remain. This fiber helps slow digestion, so the sugar does not hit your system all at once. Fruit juice you buy at the store retains all the sugar but none of the fiber and far fewer of the phytonutrients, so it's effectively the same as soda.

Dr. Barry Popkin, a professor of nutrition from the University of North Carolina at Chapel Hill, sums up the evidence about store-bought fruit juice: "From our long-term, huge studies in Singapore, Australia, the United States and Europe, I think 100 percent fruit juice is as bad as sugar-sweetened beverages for its effects on our health."

PROTEIN POWDER

So what about drinking protein? As discussed in Chapters 1 and 2, Americans already get more than enough protein, so there probably isn't a need to consume protein-based drinks.

That said, a lot of people—including the two of us—feel like having a protein-rich shake boosts our mood, gives us energy throughout the day, and is simply a great practice. Bruce has tended to be somewhat dismissive of protein powder; nevertheless, he starts every day with a fairly high-protein smoothie. If you don't want to include fortified soy milk and nuts in your smoothie, then use protein powder as Kathy does; it is another excellent option.

Be careful when shopping. Before you reach for that giant tub labeled PROTEIN, look for the ingredients. Be sure to avoid whey and casein (the overwhelming source for most protein powder), and stick with plant-based sources such as peas, rice, soy, and hemp. Whey and casein proteins are derived from dairy milk. Recall from Chapter 2 that animal protein is linked to a host of ailments, and it is impossible to isolate harmful ingredients from healthy ones. If you use whey and casein protein powder, you could be blending in problems to your otherwise healthy shake.

Animal protein powders also may contain pesticides, dioxins, and other harmful chemicals from food fed to the animals. Remember that animals have to eat many times the calories in the form of feed as we get back from any products distilled from their flesh or milk. And a lot of harmful chemicals are not water soluble, so they collect inside the animals, including the protein that becomes protein powder. So it's not surprising that when *Consumer Reports* looked at animal-based protein powders, it found that several had concerning levels of arsenic, cadmium, or lead. All of these chemicals are linked to health problems, from less serious problems like aggressive behavior and constipation to more serious diseases like brain degeneration and cancer.

So if you are going to consume protein powder, be sure to seek out brands that are plant based. The most popular plant-based protein powders are soy based, and the science indicates that soy performs similarly to animal-based proteins but without the link to cancer and other diseases. One study from the American College of Sports Medicine finds that for elite athletes, soy protein worked just as well as animal-based varieties.

The popular website bodybuilding.com points out that "soy protein has unique benefits for exercising adults in improving anti-oxidant status. These findings indicate that soy protein can help combat free radical formation during exercise, which may help speed muscle recovery after exercise." The site also mentions another advantage for soy: "In addition, soy protein consumption may provide additional health benefits including a reduced risk of coronary heart disease when combined with a healthy diet. Recent studies also demonstrate that soy protein consumption may reduce the risk of certain kinds of cancer including prostate cancer."

Another popular option for plant-based protein powder is pea protein, which digests much more easily than animal protein powders do and helps you avoid the bloating and gas that often accompanies whey and casein powder. Pea protein appears to have many of the same advantages as soy protein, most notably that it's not animal protein and therefore contains fiber, complex carbohydrates, and other nutrients. And pea protein actually has more protein when compared to whey protein, clocking in at 25 to 30 grams per scoop, compared to roughly 23 grams for most whey protein brands.

There are also new protein powders that are being made with microalgae, such as spirulina and chlorella. These are complete proteins that include fiber, vitamins, and a variety of micronutrients that you don't get in any other protein powder. Right now, the prices for microalgae are high, but if they catch on, economies of scale should allow them to one day compete with traditional protein powders. As an added benefit, microalgae uses even less fertilizer per calorie when compared to legumes, never contains pesticides, and can recirculate water in a closed system, cutting down on water needs.

CHAPTER 9

The Next Great American Meat Company

The way that we're producing meat today, using animals as the technology for turning plant biomass into meat, is the most destructive technology on earth today by a wide margin. It's a technology that was brilliant 10,000 years ago, but is completely unsuited to a world where there are billions of people who want those foods.

—PAT BROWN, FOUNDER AND
CEO OF IMPOSSIBLE FOODS

A few years back, a bunch of plant-based meat and egg companies came together for a taste-testing event for potential investors. The most famous person in the room, Bill Gates, was blown away by the plant-based chicken from Beyond Meat—the company's first product, which was developed with assistance from Whole Foods Market. He wrote about the experience in his blog, declaring, "What I was experiencing was more than a clever meat substitute. It was a taste of the future of food."

In early 2016, at the Milken Global Summit, Eric Schmidt—Board Chair of Google parent company Alphabet—was asked to reflect on six technological innovations that he believes would improve life by an order of magnitude (a factor of at least ten, meaning 1,000 percent). Schmidt discusses mostly what you'd expect from someone with his background: 3D printers for infrastructure, watches that monitor our health and alert a nearby hospital if we're about to have a heart attack, self-driving cars, and so on. But the very first tech innovation he mentioned? Plant-based meat.

Gates and Schmidt are excited about plant-based alternatives for their capacity to offer everything that consumers like about meat by using plants, thereby eliminating the harms to humans, to animals, and to the planet associated with dirty protein. With these ideals in mind, the Good Food Institute (GFI), which Bruce founded and where he serves as executive director and where Kathy serves on the board of directors, was created to promote plant-based meat and meat grown through cellular agriculture, also known as "clean meat"—more on that in the next chapter.

Animal, environmental, and health-care nonprofits have been encouraging a shift away from animal agriculture for decades. Nevertheless, meat consumption has gone up dramatically since that time, while the number of vegetarians has barely budged. Remarkably, despite hundreds of books and millions of views of horrific undercover slaughter videos, the percentage of the US population that is vegetarian sits stubbornly at 2 percent. That's what it was ten years ago, twenty years ago, thirty years ago, and so on.

We should take a step back and make two quick points: first, rates of self-identified vegetarians and people experimenting with vegetarianism are both way up from ten years ago, which is why you probably thought that actual vegetarianism is up. The problem is that most self-identified vegetarians eat meat: when research and analysis nonprofit Faunalytics asked consumers whether they had consumed chicken, pork, or fish over the past month, only 2 percent said no. Second, Faunalytics also found that more than 80 percent of people who try vegetarianism go back to eating meat.

A few comments on these two things: first, we don't care if people who eat mostly vegetarian or vegan want to call themselves vegetarian or vegan. It's like that Mark Twain line about how quitting smoking is easy—"I've done it a thousand times"—but that's okay. If people want to self-identify that way, then go for it. We also don't see value in "educating" (i.e., lambasting) people for not being sufficiently plant based; that's not going to win hearts and minds.

Second, we're not saying that education and consumer choice based on health or ethics are worthless. For examples of when education has resulted in significant changes in buying habits, just look at the "pink slime" controversy (an entire segment of the beef industry was destroyed), the collapse of the veal industry in response to consumer outrage over the treatment of calves, or the radical shift in the number of people who smoke. Indeed, both of us and many of our friends have transformed the way we eat because of education campaigns, and although 2 percent of the population is comparatively small, it's still millions of people who do not eat meat, thereby lessening the food sector's contribution to chronic disease, climate change, pollution, global poverty, animal cruelty, and countless other issues.

But even if education and ethics can transform society, we've been working at both for a very long time; perhaps we should try something different, as a complement to education. And that's where plant-based meat comes in.

The idea of creating meat from plants excites Gates, Schmidt, and many other investors in plant-based meat companies, and it's why GFI was formed: to create the products and nurture companies that will compete with animal food on taste, price, and convenience. If you were to stand outside a restaurant and poll people, you would find that everyone looks at the price and everyone thinks about the taste. And, of course, if the product is not there, people will not buy it.

We are also very glad to see how many people are participating in the slow-food movement and other efforts to improve food integrity. And we are always heartened when we see polls indicating an increased concern for the environmental consequences of food, the effect on animal welfare, and so on. But, at the end of the day, 80 percent of Americans eat fast food every single month, and half eat fast food on a weekly basis. Polls going back more than a decade have found that more than 95 percent of Americans claim they care about the treatment of farm animals, and yet at least 96 percent of Americans continue to eat factory-farmed meat.

The theory of Gates and Schmidt is that once plant-based meat tastes exactly like animal-based meat (or better) and is price competitive, it should be able to replace a huge segment of the meat industry. Something similar to this happened with plant-based milk, which twenty years ago was well under 1 percent of the milk market, but which today is roughly 10 percent of the market. Of course, few people shifted toward plant-based milk because of ethical concerns. They shifted because plant-based milks taste great and are priced competitively. Recently, General Mills filed a patent application for creating dairy-free products using chickpeas and other legumes. The burgeoning success of soy-, almond-, and other plant-based milks continues to prove that we don't need an exact replica for people to make the switch.

With sales under $500 million annually, plant-based meat is where plant-based milk was twenty years ago, though it's up against a meat sector that rakes in $200 *billion*. When plant-based meat closes that proportionality gap, it will have grown by almost 4,000 percent, which will cut climate change emissions from livestock, free up crops, and take more than a billion animals out of production agriculture.

MOVERS AND SHAKERS IN
THE NEW MEAT INDUSTRY

The plant-based meat industry is being revolutionized by two Browns: Ethan Brown and Pat Brown (no relation). Both Browns came to plant-based meat because of their concerns about climate change. Ethan received his MBA from Columbia and went to work trying to right the world by working on clean energy. When he came across the information about the impact of animal agriculture on our environment, he was shocked to his core and completely changed his focus, founding Beyond Meat in 2009. With significant support from Whole Foods and its plant-based CEO, John Mackey, Ethan worked with food scientists from the University of Missouri, which led to their launching Beyond Meat's first product in 2012: the chicken strips that wowed Bill Gates. As production scaled up, they launched in Whole Foods stores nationwide in April 2013.

Ethan has set an ambitious goal worthy of the Silicon Valley "We can do anything" mind-set that has funded his business: to decrease global meat consumption by 25 percent over the next ten years. He is on a powerful trajectory: in 2013, Ethan had products in 350 stores; within a few years, they were in more than 10,000 stores, and he had former McDonald's president Don Thompson on his board and Honest Tea founder Seth Goldman as his board's executive chair. As Ethan explains to Nicholas Kristof of the *New York Times*, "We want to create the next great American meat company. . . . That's the dream."

Pat Brown, meanwhile, had been teaching biochemistry at Stanford University, and he decided to take his 2009 sabbatical and focus on what he could do to combat climate change. After researching the issue, he came to the same conclusion as Ethan: the biggest problem was the meat industry, and the best solution was to create competing, clean protein products. And so in 2011, Pat founded Impossible Foods. Famously, Google Ventures tried to buy Impossible Foods outright, reportedly offering $300 million. Pat turned them down because he was worried that Google would not bring the same passion to the endeavor that he would. He recognized that for Google Ventures, $300 million was not that much money; a few false starts could lead the company to shut down operations. Pat was not going to let his mission-based company fail that way, even if it meant turning down $300 million. Besides, he has bigger aspirations, as he tells the German magazine *Der Spiegel* in February 2017: "We fully intend to be producing 100 percent of the ground beef in the world within the next decade or so."

Indeed, both Browns' bullishness on plant proteins has been backed by independent research. The well-respected technology research firm Lux Research predicted that plant-based meat would account for one-third of the global meat market by 2054, growing at a combined adjusted growth rate of 9 percent annually over the next forty years, against 1 percent growth for animal-based meat. Both Pat and Ethan Brown argue that we can do much better than that with the sort of backing that we have been seeing in recent years; if the plant-based meat sector were to grow at a rate of just 20 percent per year, there would be no meat industry by 2050.

We have to mention, of course, that there are other superstar plant-based meat companies that have been actively paving the way, such as the Canadian-based Gardein started by Yves Potvin more than twenty-five years ago, whose products are in more than 20,000 stores across North America. Potvin is considered to be the first to scale up a large-scale production of nonanimal meats. Chef David Lee launched Field Roast in 1997, which sprang from his nonprofit FareStart. Tofurky, Boca, Lightlife, Hungry Planet, and Morningstar are also filling out the accelerating market with excellent products.

When Bruce gives speeches, one of his favorite slides begins with this quote from former Pinnacle Foods CEO Robert Gamgort, who explains why his multibillion-dollar food conglomerate had just paid more than $150 million for Gardein: "Plant-based meats are in the early stages of a macro trend, similar to the way soy and almond milk changed the milk category." Gamgort suggests that plant-based meat is about to explode in sales, from under $500 million to over $20 billion. But Bruce's favorite part about the quote was that it came from the CEO of the company that brought us Hungry Man TV dinners and Armour potted meat.

And it's not just Pinnacle that's moved into plant-based meat. Big Food is responding to the potential to make boatloads of money in this market sector. It understands that these brands are excellent investments in both the short and long term. It's not surprising that Kellogg's, which was founded by one of the most famous vegetarians of his day, Will Keith Kellogg, owns Morningstar and Gardenburger. But it's more interesting that Kraft Foods, which also owns Oscar Mayer, purchased Boca Burger, the hottest veggie burger of its day—served by Oprah on her show and, of course, wolfed down by a certain former president.

One of our favorite stories about plant-based meat we heard from Seth Tibbott, the founder of Tofurky and one of the most kindhearted and community-minded people we have ever met. According to Seth, legend has it that Boca Burger sent a pallet of Boca Burgers to the Clinton White House that was not ordered. The White House kitchen, assuming no one would send an entire pallet of product unless it had been ordered, signed for it and took it in. Boca then immediately put out the story that "Bill Clinton loves Boca Burgers," only to get a call from the head of the US Navy, who oversees the White House kitchen, saying in very strong terms that what the president eats in the White House is classified information, and also that the president cannot endorse a brand. Boca was told to cease and desist marketing its product as "Bill Clinton's favorite meal," under some unclear penalty (Guantanamo Bay?). Of course by then the marketing machine had already done its work, and the connection had been made.

To keep up the trend of the food industry noting the promise of alternatives to animal agriculture, international food conglomerate Monde Nissin purchased plant-based meat maker Quorn for $832 million in 2015, and international dairy giant Danone purchased White Wave Foods—of Silk soy dairy alternatives fame—for more than $10 billion in 2016. Perhaps most encouraging, Tyson Foods, the largest meat company in the United States, bought a 5 percent stake in Beyond Meat in fall of 2016. Shortly after the purchase, Bruce penned an op-ed in the *Wall Street Journal* in which he celebrates Tyson Foods' decision to move into the plant-based meat sector. He also mentioned the purchase of Boca Burger by the food conglomerate Kraft Foods, which subsequently created a massive advertising budget for Boca's products, including full-page ads in *People* and *Time* as well as placement in just about every grocery store in the country.

Activity is even hotter in the venture capital world. Beyond Meat has attracted investments from Bill Gates, Twitter founders Ev Williams and Biz Stone, and one of the hottest venture capitalist firms in the world, Kleiner Perkins. Gates is also invested in Pat Brown's Impossible Foods, alongside Google Ventures, Khosla Ventures, and the richest person in Asia, Li Ka-shing. There are other powerful examples, from Salesforce founder Marc Benioff's investments in plant-based egg giant Hampton Creek and plant-based seafood startup New Wave Foods to private-equity mastermind Jeremy Coller's investments in some of the most exciting new companies, such as synthetic collagen company Gelzen, plant-based dairy company Kite Hill, and synthetic dairy company Perfect Day.

Bill Gates notes in a blog video that 92 percent of plant proteins have not yet been explored for their capacity to be turned into plant-based meat. As just one example, only ten years ago no one would have thought of pea protein as a viable option for plant-based meat; now it's the hottest option for both meat and dairy, being the primary ingredient in Beyond Meat's signature products and Ripple Foods' plant-based milk.

We know from GFI scientists that other grains have tremendous promise, including rice, oats, flax, canola, and lupin. Indeed, lupin is the primary ingredient in products from a Dutch company called the Vegetarian Butcher, whose foods are meeting with glowing reviews. Notably, lupin is a feed crop that can grow anywhere. We can easily imagine new plant-based meat companies springing up, planting their fields of lupin adjacent to the factories that will be churning out amazing plant-based meats.

———————

Bruce likes to tell the story of how he was speaking to a group of slow-food devotees at a conference called "Change Food." The title of his talk was "Markets and Food Technology Will Save the World," and he was the only person among about a dozen speakers who discussed anything other than slow, organic, grass-fed, and the like. After he spoke, people came up to him to ask him about regenerative agriculture and grass-fed beef, and a few different people mentioned enjoying veggie burgers but wanted them to taste more like vegetables, rather than trying to emulate meat.

A few days later, Bruce gave four talks over two days at Harvard's law school, business school, government school, and on the undergraduate campus. All four talks were packed with students, not one of whom asked a question that indicated concern about processing or a desire to consume products that were more vegetable based and less meat-like. Not one. Bruce has spoken many times about food technology at all of the top universities, and concern about food technology almost never comes up other than at conferences specifically dedicated to food.

And this makes sense. Recall that according to Gallup, 80 percent of Americans eat fast food at least once per month, and almost half eat fast food at least weekly. These foods tend to be some of the least sustainably produced and most damaging to public health, but people are not thinking about that when eating at McDonald's or KFC. People are choosing fast food because it's tasty, cheap, and convenient. Think also about recent predictions that global meat demand is set to grow by 20 percent in the next ten years and by more than three-quarters by the middle of the century. So although we will be thrilled if plant-based meat companies fail because consumers are so enamored of whole plant foods, we do see plant-based meat as a superb alternative to animal-based meat. And no matter how processed plant-based meat is, it will still be healthier and better for the environment than animal-based meat.

Dr. Greger once compared popular plant-based chicken from the company Gardein Foods to traditional chicken and found that plant-based chicken has half the calories, one-fourth the fat, and three times as much iron. It also has no cholesterol, no saturated fat, and a significant amount of fiber. Traditional chicken, as we know, is loaded with saturated fat and cholesterol, while containing no fiber at all. And Gardein's plant-based chicken has the same amount of protein despite having half the calories.

When Dr. Kim Williams, then president of the American College of Cardiology, read a paper by Dr. Caldwell Esselstyn, he "changed that day to a cholesterol-free diet, using meat substitutes commonly available in stores and restaurants for protein." Within six weeks, his LDL cholesterol level had fallen to 90. Dr. Williams then asks, "Wouldn't it be a laudable goal of the American College of Cardiology to put ourselves out of business?"

Well, Dr. Williams, Pat Brown—along with the other alternative meat pioneers—has just that intention when he says, "In twenty years, we want to be producing more than half of the world's supply of all of the foods we're getting from animals. We need to grow on that scale because the problem we're addressing is so urgent."

Not All Processed Foods Are Bad

You may have heard the oft-repeated mantra: avoid processed foods. Well, yes. Frozen pizza-wrapped corn dogs are definitely not good for you. Nor are store-bought cookies and cakes that are devoid of any useful nutrients and loaded with ingredients that are impossible to pronounce. But if you're reading this book, that's probably not your daily fare anyway.

We've heard from a lot of people that they don't want "fake" food like veggie burgers or "fakin' bacon." And that's fine, simple foods like whole grains, nuts, beans, and vegetables are great, but if you are anything like us, sometimes you enjoy the tradition of something like grilled sausage or a chicken sandwich. And there are delicious plant-based alternatives that are great for satisfying that craving.

The processing involved in creating plant-based meat does not detract from the fact that these are still incredibly healthy products, exponentially healthier than the animal-based versions. Just like wheat can be processed into 100 percent whole wheat bread or chickpeas into hummus, so too, plants like peas and soy can be processed into plant-based meat.

Animal based meat is not generally thought of as a "processed" product, but it does indeed go through significant processing that puts consumers at risk. For example, ground meat is not the meat from just a single animal, as it would have been a few decades ago. *Washington Post* journalist

continues

Not All Processed Foods Are Bad *continued*

Roberto A. Ferdman set out to determine how many cows go into a burger, but no one could tell him. One thing that became clear in his research, though, is that each patty is likely to contain the meat from more than one hundred different animals—which exponentially adds to the likelihood of dangerous bacterial contamination. Like we mentioned in Chapter 3, research from Johns Hopkins University found the active ingredients in Prozac and Benadryl in most of the chicken they tested. And in study after study, researchers find potentially lethal bacteria on most of the meat that is being sold in our nation's supermarkets; as just one example, *Consumer Reports* finds that 97 percent of tested raw chicken breasts were contaminated.

And even beyond the potential bacterial and chemical residues, there is a long list of approved chemicals that are used to treat meat in the United States, most designed to either kill pathogens or ensure that meat—which, after all is a carcass—from going rancid and turning a deeply unappetizing and gross-appearing gray color. Some of these additives are innocuous, but some of them are concerning.

For example, nonorganic chicken in the United States is drenched in chemicals before shipping that include chlorine, which is not allowed in most of the world and which is dangerous to both workers and chicken consumers. At animal processing factories, machines drench the carcasses in chlorinated water because of the high rates of food-borne pathogens, which, of course, is not an issue for plant-based meat. According to the *Los Angeles Times,* "Each bird can absorb 2% to 12% of its weight in this chlorinated water as it cools."

And consider what happens to a cow's milk: antibiotics are used to prevent or cure infections, and hormones are utilized to increase milk production. Too often the cow has

continues

Not All Processed Foods Are Bad *continued*

developed mastitis, a painful infection of the udders from overuse, and the milk comes out with pus or blood in it, so it's treated with antiseptics to disinfect it. There's a reason raw, unpasteurized dairy is illegal: it can be lethal. But, from where we sit, pasteurized blood and pus may not be dangerous, but it's still blood and pus (yuck)—and it's also unnatural, the product of aggressive milking protocols that cause dairy cows to give about ten times as much milk as their babies would naturally suckle. No wonder these poor animals are worn out.

Back to meat alternatives: it's true that a common additive in processing is sodium. So if you have hypertension or your doctor has told you to cut down on sodium for some other reason, check the labels of whatever food you're eating.

Things like white flour and white rice remove almost all of the phytonutrients and fiber, making them much less healthy than whole foods, true enough; but they are not harmful in themselves—they are just not as healthy as their whole food counterparts.

With plant-based meat, some phytochemicals and fiber are removed in processing, but it still has a lot of fiber and a lot of phytonutrients, where animal-based meat has no fiber and very few phytochemicals.

Lastly, plant-based meat has none of the cholesterol and problematic protein of animal-based meat, and it's generally much lower in saturated fat. It also does not present the same risk of potentially lethal bacteria, chlorine, or other chemicals as animal-based meat. The takeaway is that although plant-based meat will have a bit less fiber and more sodium than unprocessed legumes, processed plant-based meats are still far healthier than animal-based meats. As Dr. Michael Greger explains, "What chicken lacks in fiber, it makes up for in mutagenic toxins and arsenic."

Here's a chart to help you weigh the differences, so that you can decide for yourself what kind of processing you feel okay about:

Animal vs. Plant-Based Meat	Animal-Based Meat	Plant-Based Meat
Harmful Components	Animal protein, cholesterol, saturated fat, dangerous bacteria, drug and other chemical residues	No animal protein or cholesterol, generally very low in saturated fat, no bacterial or drug residues
Missing Nutrients	Zero fiber, zero complex carbohydrates, very low in phytochemicals	High in fiber, complex carbohydrates, and phytochemicals

But is it Natural?

Some people use processing as shorthand for "unnatural"—consider Michael Pollan's food rule, "Don't eat anything that your grandmother would not recognize as food." While modern meat looks like the meat of past generations, it would be hard to imagine something less natural than the way modern farms and slaughterhouses operate, what with the drugs required to keep the animals alive in putrid conditions. There is nothing natural about Prozac-dosed chickens or hormone-laced cattle feed.

And farm animals also no longer raise families, copulate naturally, or even go outside to breathe the fresh air. Their genetics have been so thoroughly manipulated that, as just one example, the upper bodies of chickens now grow more than six times as quickly as they did in our grandparents' day. Fat content has skyrocketed and death rates from lung collapse, heart failure, and crippling deformities are astronomical. There is nothing natural about the industrial farming of animals.

CHAPTER 10

Growing Meat

Growing meat from cell cultures rather than from actual living livestock could mean all types of powerful changes to industrial agriculture. We wouldn't need pesticide-laden GM corn, industrial slaughterhouses, or gasoline, because we wouldn't be feeding, slaughtering, or shipping animals around the country. We also wouldn't need to deal with the mountains (or lakes) of animal waste that contaminate our water, or clouds of methane that contribute to climate change. And we wouldn't need to kill billions of animals to satisfy our bottomless desire for protein.

—Professor McKay Jenkins, *Food Fight: GMOs and the Future of the American Diet*

When people say they can't cut out meat because they "crave" it, some might question their willpower. But that isn't fair.

As journalist Marta Zaraska discusses in *Meathooked*, there does appear to be something in either human physiology or human psychology that causes many of us to desperately want to eat meat. Perhaps it's learned and can be unlearned. Or maybe some people are hardwired to eat meat. After all, there must be a reason why so many people return to meat after trying to go plant based.

In the previous chapter we explored companies that were recreating the meat experience using plants. But for people who genuinely can't give up meat, what if there were a way to eat real meat . . . without animals?

While we share Bill Gates's and Eric Schmidt's enthusiasm for plant-based meat, we think the analogues will take us only so far. Enter "clean meat," which is produced by growing meat in what will eventually look like meat breweries. Right now, to create meat, we have to feed animals vast quantities of corn, soy, grain, and other feedstocks; this causes the animals' cells to multiply and grow, creating meat. As discussed in Chapter 3, animals are extremely inefficient in converting the energy from their feed into meat. For "clean meat," we bypass the live animals. We take a few cells from an animal and feed them with nutrients directly, causing them to multiply and grow in large tanks. It will take a fraction of the time and resources, and cause a fraction of the pollution of our current method of deforesting land to grow massive amounts of crops to feed animals, then transporting these animals to slaughter. And what we get in these meat breweries is pure meat, with no antibiotic or other drug residues and no bacterial contamination.

We call this meat "clean" instead of "cultured meat," "lab-grown meat," or "tissue-engineered meat." First, it's just wrong to call it "laboratory meat," because, once it's commercialized, it will be grown in a factory, not a lab. (Imagine if the term "factory farm" can one day mean a good thing!) Of course, all processed food starts in a food lab, but we don't refer to "lab-created corn flakes," and so on. It's also not "synthetic" meat; this is real meat just grown in a different way. Second, contaminated meat and eggs in the United

States causes tens of millions of food-borne illnesses annually and hospitalizes tens of thousands; in contrast, clean meat removes the filth of factory farms and slaughterhouses and offers consumers a much safer product.

It's also clean in the same way that "clean energy" is clean—it requires one-third the energy input of chicken (the most efficient meat) and causes a small fraction of the climate change, among a variety of other environmental benefits. According to estimates from Memphis Meats, the first private company set up to commercialize clean meat, the process of producing meat from cells will require about three caloric inputs for each caloric output. And according to research from Oxford University, clean meat production will produce about 95 percent less greenhouse gases than conventional meat.

At the Good Food Institute, senior scientist Dr. Liz Specht points out that both of those numbers are wildly preliminary, and she suggests that the real caloric conversion and climate change numbers are likely to prove even better as the technology becomes more efficient.

Many of our good friends in the food movement will argue that we should focus only on promoting a plant-based diet. In many ways, clean meat is aimed at the least common denominator: meat for the 98 percent of the population that focuses its food choices almost exclusively on price, taste, and convenience. We're completely in support of all efforts aimed at convincing consumers to consider ethics in their food purchasing decisions—we've both been doing exactly that for decades—but we're also realistic: many consumers simply won't. Clean meat is a solution for them because it makes their default choice of meat also a humane and sustainable choice. As we see it, clean meat will probably not compete with plant-based meat or a whole foods plant-based diet; clean meat will compete with factory-farmed meat.

CLEAN MEAT PIONEERS

Clean meat had its coming out party in the summer of 2013 when Dr. Mark Post grilled up a clean meat burger at a media event in central London. The price tag—roughly $1.2 million per pound, paid for by Google founder Sergey Brin, who wanted to find a better way to make meat. Since his famous burger grilling, Post has joined with former food industry executive Peter Verstrate to form a clean meat company, Mosa Meats.

Post is a top tissue-engineering scientist who has both a PhD in pharmacology and a medical degree. He taught at Dartmouth Geisel School of Medicine for ten years and Harvard Medical School for seven before being lured back to the Netherlands to teach tissue engineering and vascular physiology at one of the top medical schools in the world. Dr. Post is a good example of why we're so excited about clean meat; the man could be doing just about anything, but he's pursuing clean meat science because he sees it as a solution to some of the world's biggest problems.

A few years after Post grilled up his burger, Dr. Uma Valeti decided to launch a clean meat company, at almost precisely the same moment as Post's founding of Mosa Meats. Having witnessed animal slaughter up close as a child in India, Valeti became a committed vegetarian early in life. Years later, he would become a cardiologist at the Mayo Clinic and then in association with the University of Minnesota. While he was at Mayo, he learned about how muscle regenerates, and he performed procedures that involved injecting stem cells into patients' hearts to help the muscle grow. That triggered an aha! moment in which he thought, "Why couldn't we do this with animal meat? Why can't we grow meat outside the animal?"

Valeti discovered the nonprofit clean meat research organization New Harvest, joined the board, and eventually invited tissue engineer and clean meat scientist Nicholas Genovese to join him at the University of Minnesota. Both men quickly realized that the goal of commercialization could be reached more quickly if they moved from academia to the private sector, and Memphis Meats was born. At the time, Valeti thought, "Look, I've been thinking about this since I was twelve. I have a phenomenal career that I've been building in cardiology, but there are 35,000 cardiologists in the United States and not a single company focused on making better meat. I decided that I wanted to assemble a team and start a company."

Valeti has an impressive résumé. He trained for four years as a cardiology fellow at the Mayo Clinic and spent seven years as a tenured professor of medicine at the University of Minnesota. He served on the Board of Governors of the American College of Cardiology and as president of the Minnesota chapter of the American Heart Association. All of this served him well as he said goodbye to medicine and ventured into the world of making meat.

Two years later, Dr. Valeti's team at Memphis Meats created a meatball that cost $18,000 per pound, and, by the time the held a taste-testing event at their "farm" near San Francisco on March 14, 2017, they had the price down to less than $2,400 per pound—so less than 1 percent of what clean meat cost to produce roughly three years earlier. Expensive, yes, but note that the first iPhone cost $3.4 billion. Dr. Post and Dr. Valeti are convinced that if adequately funded, clean meat will cost less than conventional meat within a decade.

Clean meat will never prove as efficient as plant-based meat, which requires just 1 calorie of input to create 1 calorie of output. Plant-based meat will also win the health competition. Americans are already consuming too much animal protein and the ills that come along for the ride, from saturated fat to the carcinogens that are created with cooking. Clean meat will still have these problems at least initially, though Post and Valeti are both committed to solving them eventually. But, perhaps most impressively, the issue of massive ecological damage will be solved. Solved also would be the problem of feeding an increasingly wealthy and populous world that craves meat. And of course the horrendous problem of how animals are raised and slaughtered for food would be eliminated. Not only could clean meat be its own multibillion-dollar business, but because it's going to be cheaper and far more sustainable than animal food as we know it today, it just might also save the planet.

The question remains, Will the average person embrace clean meat? We think so. Recall that right now, people eat meat *despite* how it's produced, not *because* of how it's produced. Most don't think about the inefficiency, the disgusting conditions on factory farms and in factory slaughterhouses, or the cruelty. Once there is an alternative that is healthier, doesn't include the filth, and doesn't harm animals, we suspect that people will, indeed, opt for the cleaner version.

There is nothing to hide in the making of clean meat, whereas there is much to hide in the process of turning animals into food. Slaughterhouses don't let cameras in because they don't want consumers to see what goes on inside. But, as we write, there are four clean meat companies—Post's, Valeti's, and two in Israel, Super-Meat and Meat the Future, which already have investment from the biggest conventional meat company in Israel—and all four of them are talking about live-streaming their operations on the Internet. We are aware of at least two more companies that plan to launch soon, and there is elevated interest among academic tissue engineers across the world. This level of interest stems in large part from an innate discomfort with the way that meat is made currently, and we take the commitment to transparency as a good sign for the future.

Not long ago, Bruce delivered a presentation at the MIT Sloan School of Management about the tantalizing possibilities of plant-based and clean meat. After the talk, he said to the audience of about a hundred students, "As you just heard, meat is made up of lipids, amino acids, minerals, and water. Researchers are quickly closing in on the creation of plant-based meat that tastes identical to chicken, has the exact same mouthfeel, and is identical in all perceptible ways. Once we have this product, plant-based meat, and once it's cheaper, would you be willing to shift your meat consumption from actual animals to plant-based meat? Please raise your hand if you would."

Most hands were raised, but nowhere near all of them.

Then he said, "As you also just heard, other researchers are using standard tissue engineering techniques to grow real meat in what will basically look like giant meat fermenters. Once at scale, this will be the exact same product—identical to conventional meat in every way, but cleaner. Once we have this product and once it's cheaper, would you be willing to shift your meat consumption from conventional meat to clean meat? Please raise your hand if you would."

Almost everyone raised their hands.

Our goal is to replicate the success of plant-based milk, where about 90 percent of plant-based milk consumers are also purchasing animal-based milk. In the short term, we are not aiming for everyone to switch exclusively to plant-based or clean meat. As we discussed in the previous chapter, we hope meat-eaters will opt to consume plant-based meat as an alternative to animal-based meat as often as possible. Nevertheless, that so many MIT graduate students in management—well educated, young, health conscious— would happily switch to clean meat but not to plant-based meat served as a wake-up call and an indication of how much people want to eat the meat of animals.

Even Lisa Keefe, an editor of *Meatingplace,* the magazine for North American beef, pork, and poultry processors, suggests that the meat industry should "see protein production less as an agricultural issue and more as a technology issue," just as Silicon Valley investors do. She specifically flagged clean meat as a possibility for either research and development or for acquisition.

Dan Murphy of *Meat Marketing & Technology*, who founded *Meatingplace* in 1996 after serving as vice president for public affairs at the meat industry's flagship lobbying group, the American Meat Institute, seems to agree. In a column for Drover's Cattle Network (slogan: "Driving the Beef Market"), he mentions that "a significant percentage of the nation's cattle, dairy and feed crop production are currently dependent on the irrigation water drawn from the Ogallala Aquifer," which is "increasingly being depleted beyond any possible replenishment."

He then posits, "an option that must be seriously considered"— clean meat—and concludes by asking, "What happens when the depletion of the Ogallala Aquifer isn't a future projection but a here-today reality? What do we do when irrigation sources elsewhere . . . no longer support the level of farm productivity we've come to depend upon? I'm not sure if the solution is deployment of massive bioreactors producing . . . animal-free meat, but it sure isn't an option that ought to be dismissed."

When you have the editor of *Meatingplace* and meat industry veteran Dan Murphy looking toward clean meat, can the meat industry itself be far behind? Apparently not. Tyson food scientist Hultz Smith appeared at a panel discussing the technology in the fall of 2016 and expressed support, and Kevin Myers, who serves as vice president for research and development at Hormel Foods, told the *Wall Street Journal* that the company sees clean meat as "a good long-term proposition." Myers has been a meat industry food scientist for more than twenty-five years, previously at Oscar Mayer and for the past fifteen years at Hormel.

Perhaps the most interesting move to date has been the launch by Tyson Foods of a $150 million fund that will, according to its press release, "focus on the areas of alternative proteins, elimination of food waste and leveraging innovative trends in technology." When asked by the *Wall Street Journal* whether these "alternative proteins" would include clean meat, Tyson confirmed that, yes, clean meat was among the technologies that Tyson would be exploring.

You might want to think of it this way: flash back to 1894, and there were almost 200,000 horses in New York City, and millions in cities across the globe. In New York, these horses were excreting 50,000 tons of manure every month. The streets were disgusting: flies, rotting carcasses, and massive piles of manure around every corner. In 1898, the first urban planning conference was convened, and the only item on the agenda was what to do about all of the horse waste that was breeding disease in cities across the Western world. But the conveners couldn't figure it out; they saw no solution, and they all went home demoralized. Flash forward just ten years to 1908, and Henry Ford debuts the Model T. By 1912, there were more cars than horses in New York, and what had been seen as an insoluble problem was solved.

We are convinced that in the same way it would be absurd for us to travel from Los Angeles to New York City on horseback, it will one day be considered absurd to grow crops, feed those crops to animals, raise those animals, ship those animals to slaughterhouses, and slaughter those animals, when we can get the exact same product in a much easier and cleaner way.

For the new generation of concerned protein consumers, this can't happen quickly enough.

PART 3

Put Clean Protein into Action

CHAPTER 11

How to Shop

You might be thinking, wait, how hard can it be to shop? And it's not. But it takes a minute to pivot from your usuals and start stocking your fridge and pantry with foods that fall in line with your fresh, clean outlook. Where it used to be a perusal through the animal-meat/butcher section of the grocery store for protein, now you'll be loading up black beans and lentils, wild mushrooms, alternative meats, and a bunch of other delicious animal-free foods into your cart. It's actually kind of fun to start planning the meals you're going to have, and a few little organizational tools will keep things easy.

For some food, it's just a matter of sidestepping. This is especially easy with dairy products: instead of cow's milk, you can pick up the hottest new plant-based milk, Ripple (brought to you by the same team that created Method cleaning products) or one of dozens of soy, almond, cashew, rice, coconut, or hemp milks. (And many brands offer delicious blends.) Instead of butter on your morning toast, pick up Earth Balance, Miyoko's, or other plant-based spreads. If you prefer cream cheese, there are many varieties such as Kite Hill, Tofutti, or Follow Your Heart.

Once relegated to crunchy-granola health-food stores, dairy-free cheeses are now ubiquitous at Whole Foods, food co-ops, and health food stores, and you can generally find a reasonable variety in national grocers like Target, Walmart, and Safeway. Brands such as Daiya, Chao, and Treeline make products that taste impossibly close to the cow variety. As for entertaining, wine with Kite Hill or Miyoko's nut-based cheese is a sure bet, while Punk Rawk and Heidi Ho are excellent plant-based cheese spreads. If you're a yogurt fan, you might want to pick up a large size of Kite Hill unsweetened plain; you can make sauces with it, or mix fruit and nuts into it for a snack or light meal. There are so many great protein powders, but, again, be careful to avoid dairy-based whey or casein; opt for plant-based varieties such as Vega or Sun Warrior. Store brands that feature pea or soy protein usually taste great, too.

From high-protein chickenless nuggets to veggie bacon strips to amazingly good veggie hot dogs, there are healthy, clean alternatives to just about every traditional animal food. Love your desserts? Thanks to a petition that received more than 28,000 signatures, Ben & Jerry's is now making dairy-free versions of its most popular flavors using coconut and almond milk. We love So Delicious, Almond Dream, Luna and Larry's, and Tofutti, which have been plant-based from the beginning. A new favorite among the celebrity set in Los Angeles is Craig's Vegan, born from a paparazzi-stalked restaurant with patrons clamoring for something dairy-free and delicious. Coffee Mate made its first foray into a new line of coconut- and almond-based creamers. Okay, these are not the power-packed proteins you're itching to stock up with, but they're easy pivots toward foods that are free of cholesterol and other inflammatory animal products.

As you transition to clean protein, don't get bogged down with nit-picking, and focus instead on the big picture. Start looking at the labels, yes, but really the focus is to simply root out the obvious animal stuff and not worry too much about the little stuff. Think Big Picture; think long term. "Lean into it," is Kathy's mantra.

MEAL PLANNING

In planning your meals, think in terms of alternatives. . . . You can still make most of your favorite recipes with just a few substitutions. If you love taco night, simply replace the meat with Beyond Meat Beefy Crumbles, Boca Meatless Ground Crumbles, or another awesome plant-based meat (or if you want to go old school, you could use tempeh, which you can grind it up just like beef and flavor with your preferred spices and sauces, or keep it simple with black beans). Portabella mushrooms have a wonderful umami flavor and feel, and can substitute for filets of just about anything, while eggplant has a decadent, meaty taste that easily stands in for chicken cutlets. Even though neither may win awards for being the biggest sources of protein, they're meaty in texture and can be used in conjunction with other vegetables and grains to get you to your target protein intake. Try hearty pastas made with white beans and tomatoes; sushi rolls with tofu, avocado, and cucumber; cauliflower and chickpea fritters; curried tofu and plantains with rice and vegetables. Remember, the abundant fiber in these foods will help you to feel full, energized, and satisfied. Part of the protein obsession, we think, is that people want to feel like they're eating solid, substantial meals. We want to feel full, fed, and nourished. So it need not be so much about counting grams or calories, but rather how fulfilled we feel.

We love the plant-based versions of pulled pork, sausage, and all of that stuff, too. You can be a righteous health-food eater and insist on only whole foods, or you can enjoy this transition and experiment with all the wonderful options on the market these days. Is a veggie burger as good as rice and beans with kale? Maybe

not, but it's a whole lot better than the cholesterol-laden, IGF-1-
inducing, dripping-with-saturated-fat animal version. Just keep in
mind that progress rather than perfection will serve you well over
the long run.

Basically, these are your proteins (more on them below):

- Plant-based meat
- Plant-based milk
- Beans and legumes
- Quinoa
- Edamame, hummus
- Whole grains
- Nuts, nut butters, seeds
- Tofu, tempeh, seitan
- Artichokes, wild mushrooms, hearts of palm
  (meaty texture + umami flavor = satisfied belly)
- Protein powders

The thing you want to do is stock your pantry with everything
you need for the week, along with some basics for the freezer that
you can always rely on. Just like you may have had frozen chicken
wings and pork chops you could pull out at a moment's notice,
you'll instead want to have some plant-based versions that you can
whip up a meal around. The more stocked you are with animal-free
proteins—just like with meat, dairy, and eggs—the easier it is to
throw together something protein rich and satisfying. No more
opening your fridge and wondering what to eat, and no desperate
trips to the grocery store.

Here's what Kathy's fridge and freezer are always stocked with:
plant-based versions of sausage, bacon, yogurt, milk and creamer,
butter, and cheese, along with a big bag of mixed greens, various vegetables, avocados, apples, hummus, and tofu, as well as a

rotating variety of almond, peanut, and cashew butter. (Of course there are beverages, too, like coconut water and wine!) She's always got whole grain English muffins and bread for toasting or sandwiches, and, tortillas, too. Most importantly, Kathy has her favorite sauces like Sriracha, peanut- and plant-based chipotle mayo, along with creamy vegan salad dressings.

In the freezer are bags of kale, broccoli, spinach, strawberries, mangos, cherries, peeled and halved bananas for smoothies, pizza crusts, veggie burger and "chick'n" patties, and prepackaged hors d'oeuvres like "chicken fingers" that can be quickly cooked in a toaster oven. There's an entire section reserved for left-over thick bean soups. And nondairy ice-cream! The pantry stores a healthy mix of whole grain pastas, canned tomatoes and pizza sauce, dried and canned beans of at least five varieties, rice, quinoa, and steel-cut oats, whole grain crackers and tortilla chips, and plant-based protein powder. On the countertop is a row of jars containing different kinds of nuts and seeds along with dried (unsweetened) fruit. Kathy keeps a basic list on her phone so when grocery shopping it's easy to scan and see what's needed.

Bruce and his wife Alka make sure to always have plenty of fresh fruit in their fridge and frozen fruit in their freezer; a variety of plant-based meat from Tofurky, Field Roast, and Beyond Meat; Miyoko's and Kite Hill cheeses and yogurts; plenty of fresh greens, plus summer squash in the summer and winter squash in the fall and winter; hummus and guacamole; their plant-based milk of choice used to be the 365 brand of soy milk, but they have recently switched to Ripple; white wine and a locally brewed beer; a variety of plant-based ice creams, usually including at least two Ben & Jerry's flavors; a few loaves of bread for peanut butter sandwiches; a variety of jellies and jams and other condiments; and lots of left-overs, because they cook a lot over the weekend, so that they can eat great food all week long.

Bruce has a basement that serves as a massive pantry, where he and Alka have a wide variety of grains, rice, dry beans, various canned beans (including refried beans), Hormel veggie chili, boxes of Clif Bars, various granolas and other breakfast cereals, various pastas and baked goods mixes, sweet chili Doritos (you haven't lived . . .), huge jars of mixed nuts from Costco, pasta sauces and canned tomatoes, more beer and wine, ground peanut butter from Whole Foods, a variety of packaged stuffed olives, and a variety of Indian spices and condiments.

Begin by setting aside a little time to plan your meals. What are you eating for breakfast, lunch, and dinner for each day of the week? Scan through the ingredients and write down everything you don't have stocked. Pro tip: Plan meals with as many

---

Jackfruit

Ever tried jackfruit? It might be one of the best clean foods you can add into your traditional dishes for a meaty flavor. . . . Jackfruit is a tropical fruit that you can buy frozen, dried, or canned. Because of its fleshy texture, people often mistake it for chicken or pork. It has a slightly sweet pineapple flavor and is able to absorb whatever spices and sauces you throw at it. Jackfruit is routinely used throughout Asia as a meat substitute and is cherished for its delightful taste. Try using it in tacos, wraps, sandwiches, or stir-fry! It may not be super high in protein (although it certainly has some), but it'll satisfy your craving for the meaty texture you're used to. And that counts for a lot, because we're not just talking health and environment, here, but also your enjoyment and pleasure!

overlapping ingredients as possible. This saves money and makes your shopping bags much lighter. Once all your meals are planned, your jaunt to the market will be completely painless.

Now let's take some time to plan your meals, because if you have a list and an idea of what to eat, you won't be caught hungry and frustrated. Begin by asking yourself, "What am I going to have for my protein?" Next, "What will be my carbohydrates and starches?" Finally, "What will be my veggies?" Each meal and shopping list should be planned around these three food groups, because when you combine all three, you'll have a truly satisfying and fulfilling meal—both visually and nutritionally.

PROTEIN

Since you probably grew up with protein as the center of your plate, that's probably what you'll want to continue doing so that your meals feel familiar and satisfying. After a while, you'll likely develop a taste for more heritage grains and beans, and you'll start heaping more greens into the mix. You might also move away from the standard grouping of "protein, starch, and veggies" and instead get more into mixed bowls or "family style" of shared dishes, but that will come as you get used to different fare.

When selecting your protein, stock up with products that have long shelf lives; this way you can safely buy all your food for the week. For instance, canned beans and lentils will sit happily in your pantry for years, and dried mushrooms and beans from the bin should last just as long. A sealed package of tofu or seitan will last weeks, while an opened (and refrigerated) package should be fresh for up to a week.

Remember that *every* plant food contains protein, so there is no shortage of ways to obtain the necessary amount. So let's go through this a little more. . . .

Protein Shopping List

We've talked about all of this, but just to recap so that it's all in one place:

Meat alternatives. Plant-based meats can easily be substituted for animal products. You'll also see a lot of pea protein as the base of alternative meats, because it's a high-quality, mild-tasting base for plant-based proteins. At the top of the ingredient list for most plant-based meats are grains, which are very high in protein. Although you might be tempted to have delicious veggie burgers and chickenless nuggets at the center of every meal, keep in mind they can be a tad pricy (not always, and not compared to meat, but compared to simpler whole foods). Meat alternatives are a solid choice at the beginning of your clean protein journey and may continue to be throughout your life. Some people, as they get more comfortable with plant foods, or want to eat more simply with only whole foods, may opt to base their meals on whole, plant-based ingredients that are both affordable and delicious.

This is a leaning-in process, and, as you gain more confidence in the kitchen, you'll find that you can cook your own great-tasting meat alternatives for less money than prepackaged varieties.

Beans. Beans are superfoods. They're loaded with protein, vitamins, and antioxidants that ward off cancer, heart disease, diabetes, and countless other chronic diseases. Beans (and lentils and peas) are also an excellent source of fiber, meaning you will be happily full after every meal. Keep your pantry stocked with black beans, chickpeas (great for salads!), kidney beans, black-eyed peas, pinto beans, and lentils. And if you really get into it, there are wonderful heritage and sprouted beans you can search for online or in farmers markets. You'll find that beans go well with almost any meal, from salads to grain bowls to casseroles. Pro tip: If you're cooking from scratch, soak them overnight in order to remove some of the indigestible sugars that cause gas. (You can also take Beano or some other digestive enzyme. But don't fear: it won't take long for your body to get used to beans, and the belly bloat you may or may not experience is only temporary!) Put the beans into a bowl or pot and cover with cool water. After an overnight soak (or roughly eight hours) pour off the water, and cook as instructed. If you're using canned beans, rinse off the liquid they were packed in, as it can be a salty brine that you don't need. Another reason you might be gassy at first is that your body has to adjust to the amount of healthy fiber it's getting now . . . and that's a good thing! You want a daily diet of lots of fiber so that your blood sugar remains steady and your bowel movements regular.

Nuts and seeds. Ounce for ounce, nuts and seeds may just be the healthiest food on the planet. One study found that merely eating a handful of nuts five or more days per week can extend your life by two years. Nuts and seeds crammed with protein include pumpkin seeds, squash seeds, pistachios, almonds, sunflower seeds, sesame seeds, flaxseeds, cashews, and walnuts. Eat them alone or crush them up in your favorite salad, oatmeal, or pasta dish—just about any meal you can think of. Many delicious plant-based cheeses and sauces use nuts as a base, so always be sure to buy in bulk. Nut butters are great for snacks, sandwiches, smoothies, or spoonfuls!

Flax and chia seeds are great sources not only of protein but also of the very important omega-3 fatty acids, and here's a little tip on both:

1. For flax, if you don't have a Vitamix, about twice a week, use a clean coffee grinder or food processor to grind up about a cup of flaxseeds so that the flax meal is ready

to use in smoothies, and then store it in the fridge or freezer. Why? Because the seeds are very small, it's unlikely that you'll chew them open, so if you don't mechanically grind them first, they'll just pass through your body without releasing all their nutritional goodness. Avoid buying already-ground seeds because the meal can go rancid rather quickly. High-speed blenders like Vitamix or Nutribullet are powerful enough to grind the seeds in the smoothie (regular-speed blenders might not), so it'll save you the step of grinding and storing.

2. For chia, just know that once liquid is added to them, they will quickly swell and create a thick mixture. That's great if you're making chia seed pudding, but if you don't want a vegetable or smoothie sludge, limit how much chia you add into the mix. Experiment until you find the right thickness that's pleasing to you.

Hummus and edamame are go-to snacks and are great to serve at cocktail hour, too; they're loaded with protein, fiber, and minerals.

Quinoa is excellent as a base for mixed bowls, sprinkled into salads, used as a bed for vegetables, or as a breakfast dish with nuts and dates (or whatever your fancy) stirred into it. Along with 8 grams of complete protein per cup, it's packed with other essential nutrients including fiber, manganese, phosphorous, folate, potassium, and iron. Better yet, it cooks in twenty minutes. Even though it's a seed, it tastes and feels like a grain, so we've given it its own category!

Tofu, tempeh, and seitan are the tried-and-trues that have been on the market for ages, and we wholeheartedly recommend keeping this traditional fare in your kitchen. Soy based, tofu will take on the flavor of whatever you spice it up with while tempeh has a wonderful fermented taste. (By the way, unflavored tempeh can be an acquired taste, so if at first you're not fond of it, you're not alone!) If you are lucky enough to have a Chinatown near where you live, there are a gazillion different types and textures of tofu, and we highly encourage exploring. Were you to see the tofu display in any city in China, you'd think it akin to the butchers department back here in the States; in fact, there's even more variety of the soy protein than there is animal protein here.

Although some people avoid wheat (we don't!), seitan is said to be a creation by ancient Buddhist monks who wanted to avoid meat but needed something substantial yet humble to eat. It's super high in protein (more than tofu) and has an excellent meaty taste and texture; you can melt (plant-based) cheese over it with some tomato sauce on top, and it's an upgraded and healthier version of a "veal Parmesan."

Artichokes, wild mushrooms, and hearts of palm are meaty in texture, which make excellent starters for a hearty main dish. Mushrooms, especially, have fantastic immune-boosting properties.

Whole grains are sometimes referred to as "the seeds of civilization" for good reason. They've been the foundational food of humans since the earliest of times because they're full of protein, energy-giving (good, complex) carbohydrates, minerals, and vitamins (especially B vitamins). They're high in protein, complement beans and legumes with their amino acids, and if in their natural unrefined state, they're low on the glycemic index. Steel cut oats and wheat are highest in protein, but barley, corn, rice, millet, teff, and others are all valuable in your pantry. When combined with beans or legumes over the course of the day (meaning you don't have to eat them together at one sitting) grains provide a complete source of protein, with all the necessary amino acids covered.

Protein powders are the perfect quick nutritional fix to have in smoothies, mixed into cashew or soy-based yogurt, or stirred into a pudding for a snack. Look for one sweetened with stevia if you want to keep it low on the glycemic index.

Our friends over at No Meat Athlete created an excellent chart showing what to look for when shopping for clean protein.

NO MEAT ATHLETE — BEST PLANT-BASED SOURCES OF PROTEIN

NUTS AND SEEDS

Food	Serving Size	Calories (Cal)	Protein (G)	Calories from Protein
Hemp seeds	1 oz	162	10	25%
Pumpkin seeds, kernels only	1 oz	151	7	19%
Peanuts, without shells	1 oz	164	7	17%
Black walnuts	1 oz	173	7	16%
Pistachios, without shells	1 oz	160	6	15%
Sunflower seeds	1 oz	164	6	15%
Almonds	1 oz	167	6	14%
Cashews	1 oz	155	5	13%
Flax seeds	1 oz	150	5	13%
Chia seeds	1 oz	137	4	12%
Walnuts	1 oz	185	4	9%

VEGETABLES

Food	Serving Size	Calories (Cal)	Protein (G)	Calories from Protein
Spinach, cooked	1 cup	41	5	49%
Mushrooms, cooked	1 cup	42	5	48%
Asparagus	1 cup	27	3	44%
Broccoli	1 cup	31	2.6	34%
Brussels sprouts	1 cup	38	3	32%
Peas, cooked	1 cup	134	9	27%
Kale, cooked	1 cup	36	2	22%

PROTEIN POWDER

Food	Serving Size	Calories (Cal)	Protein (G)	Calories from Protein
Soy protein	1 oz	112	24	86%
Pea protein	1 oz	103	21	83%
Spirulina	1 oz	81	16	79%
Brown rice protein	1 oz	99	18	73%
Hemp protein	1 oz	85	13	61%

BEANS AND LEGUMES

Food (cooked)	Serving Size	Calories (Cal)	Protein (G)	Calories from Protein
Tempeh	½ cup	180	16	46%
Tofu	½ cup	94	10	43%
Soy beans	½ cup	127	11	35%
Brown lentils	½ cup	115	9	31%
Red lentils	½ cup	115	9	31%
Green lentils	½ cup	115	9	31%
Kidney beans	½ cup	120	7	28%
Split peas	½ cup	116	8	28%
Lima beans	½ cup	109	7.5	28%
Cannellini beans	½ cup	100	7	28%
Navy beans	½ cup	90	6	27%
Black-eyed peas	½ cup	80	5	25%
Black beans	½ cup	100	6	24%
Pinto beans	½ cup	100	6	24%
Chickpeas (Garbanzo beans)	½ cup	120	6	20%

BREAD, GRAINS, PASTA

Food (cooked)	Serving Size	Calories (Cal)	Protein (G)	Calories from Protein
Seitan	½ cup	180	31.5	70%
Whole wheat bread	2 slices	138	7	20%
Spelt	½ cup	123	5.5	18%
Whole wheat pasta	½ cup	87	3.5	16%
Teff	½ cup	128	5	14%
Quinoa	½ cup	111	4	14%
Oats	½ cup	154	5.5	14%
Buckwheat	½ cup	284	9.5	13%

Created by No Meat Athlete (nomeatathlete.com)

HEALTHY CARBOHYDRATES

Aside from the whole grains themselves, opt for whole-grain pasta made from wheat, rice, or quinoa; these noodles will have their fiber intact. Pasta, grains, and quinoa have extremely long shelf lives, so you can buy them in bulk, which is always cheaper.

Starchy vegetables such as potatoes, roots, parsnips, pumpkin, squash, and zucchini also contain healthy carbohydrates and deserve a prominent place in your pantry. (Sweet potatoes were the go-to staple for the longest-living women in the world in Okinawa, Japan!)

Healthy Carbohydrate Shopping List

Bread. Hang on, you might be saying; this book is supposed to be about protein! But did you know that according to the Mayo Clinic, two slices of whole grain bread have about 7.2 grams of protein? Consider that one egg has only 6 grams of protein, and if you eat only the white, you're just getting 3 grams. So, given that bread has a good dose of protein inherent in the grain, you can feel great about making it the building block of a snack or light bite. Add some nut butter or hummus, and you have a healthy dose of protein!

Before you buy, check the ingredients panel to make sure there are several grams of fiber per serving. Low-quality products like white bread have little to no fiber, almost no phytonutrients, and can have a good bit of sugar and salt. Avoid products with gimmicky labels like "multigrain" or "made with whole grains." Some manufacturers will even dye their bread brown to make it look healthier, but the ingredient panel never lies. Make sure the label says "100 percent whole wheat" (or rye or oat, etc.) to ensure you are getting a quality product with its fiber and nutrients intact. Even better, look for sprouted breads made without flour.

(There's a wonderful one called Manna bread that's great to have at breakfast!) High-quality breads without artificial preservatives do go stale faster, but you can extend their freshness by refrigerating them. If your grocery store is having a sale, buy extras and store them in the freezer.

Brown rice and quinoa. The bigger the package, the lower the cost per serving. Make sure you always have these staples in your pantry. Grocers often have bulk discounts, so don't be afraid to buy big during sales. Stocking up on several months' worth of grains might seem expensive and wasteful at the time, but you save money in the long run, not to mention lighten your shopping bag for future trips. Cooked brown rice and quinoa keep for up to a week in the fridge, so you can safely seal leftovers. There are also precooked versions sold in small packages that are microwavable, making them super convenient for a quick and easy meal. In a pinch, that with a can of beans and a corn tortilla is a satisfying and protein-rich meal. Add avocado, salsa, and a big salad and you're set to impress!

Oatmeal. A perfect breakfast should be fast, delicious, and energizing, and it should keep you full until lunchtime. No small feat! Fortunately, oatmeal checks all of these boxes, and it's high on the protein scale. Oatmeal is absorbed slowly and provides your body a steady supply of energy, like a slow-burning log. Meanwhile, the fiber creates a gelling effect in your stomach that keeps you satiated all morning. Traditional unsweetened oatmeal is best, but there are quick-cook varieties that are ready in minutes; just be careful they're not chock full of sugar. Opt for steel-cut because that's the whole, unprocessed grain. Bring four parts water to a boil at night, put in one part oats, and turn off the heat and cover. By morning your oats will be fully cooked and ready to go by just heating them up. Save the leftovers for a few days of breakfasts, or make some healthy pancakes from them—there are a ton of recipes on the web. Add chopped nuts and fruit, and there's almost nothing more satisfying. If you want an extra dose of protein, add a scoop of your favorite powder to the oats just before eating (rather than mixing it in the night before). Eating more protein in the morning helps you feel satiated, and thus you're likely to consume fewer calories later in the day.

Starches. Potatoes have an unfair reputation as "empty" calories, largely because of processed foods like French fries and potato chips. Don't be fooled—potatoes are among the healthiest foods on the planet. Believe it or not, a large russet potato has about 8 grams of protein (more than the 6 in an egg, with none of the cholesterol or saturated fat), and that covers about 14 to 17 percent of your daily protein need. Top it with some baked beans or a chargrilled plant-protein patty, and you're really supercharging your numbers. Potatoes are packed with antioxidants, vitamin B6, potassium, vitamin C, and many other nutrients. In fact, scientists at the Institute for Food Research found that potato compounds called kukoamines can help lower your blood pressure. You can also buy them in bulk; potatoes last weeks in the pantry and many months in the fridge. For maximum health benefits, buy antioxidant-packed sweet potatoes. Not only arc tubers great nutritionally, but they help you feel full and satisfied.

Other ideas: couscous, noodles made from black beans, chickpeas or tofu, German black bread, whole-grain or corn tortillas.

FRUITS AND VEGETABLES

Reserve plate space for fruits and vegetables at every meal. To save money, buy fruits and veggies that are in season—more supply means lower prices. In the winter, look for Brussels sprouts, cabbage, carrots, celery, grapefruit, kale, and winter squash. In the

How to Compare Prices

Everyone wants to find the best deal at the grocery store, but it's not always easy with so many products and sizes. It might seem logical to reach for the cheapest box of brown rice, but you might actually be losing money compared to a higher-priced, yet much larger, package.

Many grocery stores have a "price per weight" label to help you compare different-sized brands. For instance, one 16-ounce package of rice might cost only $4.99 ($0.31 per ounce), but you'd be better off choosing the 32-ounce package for $6.50 ($0.20 per ounce). That's a per-ounce difference of $0.11. It may not seem like much, but other price differences can be much larger and over weeks and months can really add up, especially for products that can be stored for long periods.

If your store doesn't have this label, just use your phone's calculator to divide the price of an item by its weight. Now you can compare products of all shapes and sizes to find the best deal, every time. All of this said, shopping for clean protein should save you a lot of money that you'd normally be spending on meat and dairy. It's a myth that clean eating is more expensive; it's not, especially if you're sticking with whole, unprocessed foods. Those things are simple, and they're cheap.

spring, try bananas, collards, peas, radishes, Swiss chard, and broccoli. In the summer, opt for beets, bell peppers, eggplant, blackberries, peaches, plums, and blueberries. In the fall, cauliflower, cranberries, ginger, green beans, mangos, and mushrooms. Sticking to what's in season makes you not just a savvy shopper but a skilled cook able to handle a wide variety of foods.

In addition, avoid prepackaged fruits and vegetables. Grocers often sell plastic-sealed broccoli florets, presliced bell peppers, peeled garlic, diced onions, and chopped fruit. It might seem tempting to save a few minutes while prepping your meals, but apart from the wasteful packaging, these products are usually much more expensive. If you know you'll be in a rush, then go ahead—otherwise, you will get much more bang for your buck by buying whole fruits and vegetables. Personally, we buy big bags of the mixed greens straight from the grocery bin and use that to green up our meals all week long. We even add those greens to smoothies for an extra dose of phytonutrients!

Your local farmers market is a great opportunity to find locally grown produce and support local businesses. Buying straight from the source means your food is super fresh and therefore more nutritious. But farmers markets can also be more expensive than a grocery store. Try shopping at the end of the day when growers are willing to unload the last of their produce at a discount.

Big box stores like Costco have great deals on frozen plant-based meats, precooked whole grains, nuts and nut butters, non-dairy milks, and produce (both fresh and frozen); we tend to stock up on the basics about once a month.

And, on that last item, there's nothing wrong with frozen fruits and vegetables. Meal planning can be hectic, and last-minute plans can mean those organic blueberries go bad before you're able to eat them. You can buy frozen fruits and vegetables in bulk and not worry about them spoiling. Frozen is often cheaper than fresh, and it's actually as, if not more, nutritious. That's because frozen fruits and vegetables are frozen immediately after they are picked—locking in nutrients that are lost when fresh produce is transported long distances. If you want to avoid turning them to mush, steam the veggies on the stovetop, bringing ½ cup of water to boil in a saucepan over medium heat, or by popping them in the microwave with a little water—no more than enough to cover a third of the veggies. Cook just until they're heated through. (Start checking at two minutes.)

Because fruits and vegetables are so versatile and can be cooked in so many ways, you'd do well to always have a variety ready to go for any meal, from quick salads to dinners. Take note of any specialty ingredients when planning your meals, but you'll find that the following fruits and vegetables will be enough for the vast majority of recipes, so be sure to stock up.

Fruits and Vegetables Shopping List

Essential "everyday" veggies: lettuces, broccoli, carrots, cauliflower, celery, garlic, onions, sugar snap peas, tomatoes, cucumbers, and bell peppers. These form the basis of countless meals. They're great in soups, green smoothies, and on sandwiches. Sauté them with your favorite sauces and fill out your meals with as much color as you can. Other great options are zucchini, mushrooms, squash, and asparagus. Since you will be using these staples so often, you can buy them fresh.

Frozen vegetables. Again, it's great to have an emergency stash of frozen broccoli, asparagus, corn, peas, and cauliflower in your freezer.

Leafy greens. In your crisper, keep kale, salad greens, and spinach. These are incredibly versatile greens that fit any meal, from light breakfast toppings to lunch salads to taco bowls.

Fruit. Contrary to what some people believe, you can't have too much fruit . . . as long as you're eating the whole fruit rather than just drinking the juice. The sugar inherent in fruit is natural and is perfectly balanced by the fiber that helps release the glucose into your body. Have a wide selection of fruit in your house. Whether topping your morning oatmeal with berries, slathering peanut butter on sliced apples, garnishing your salad with pomegranate seeds, or forming the base of your smoothie, there is never a bad time to integrate healthy, delicious fruit into your meal. For basics, always keep on hand apples, bananas, and oranges, then supplement with in-season fruits. In your freezer you might want to have frozen strawberries, blueberries, pineapples, and bananas (peel them before freezing). You don't have to wait for frozen berries to thaw—you can drop them into your oatmeal or blend them up for a refreshing smoothie. And pick up some dried fruit—not only do they retain most of the micronutrients, fiber, and antioxidants of their fresh counterparts; they have very long shelf lives—opt for unsweetened.

Other ideas: canned diced tomatoes, dried mushrooms, jarred artichokes, olives, hearts of palm.

And, by all means, keep avocados on hand for sandwiches, toast, guacamole, or garnish! They're even great to make a smoothie more creamy.

Should You Buy Organic Produce?

Whenever you walk through the grocery store, you're bombarded with labels: "all natural," "fat free," and "lightly sweetened" are just a few of the gimmicky labels food manufacturers slap onto their products to fool you. In most cases there is little to no oversight over the use of healthy-sounding labels. However, organic is different.

To display the organic label, a product has to be minimally processed without synthetic preservatives or artificial ingredients and cannot be genetically modified, and there are a variety of strictures that make for much better land use and much less wild animal death.

---

continues

Should You Buy Organic Produce? *continued*

For example, farms that grow organic produce are prohib-ited from using most pesticides and must practice sustainable growing methods. As a result, organic products generally in-volve a lot less accidental poisoning of animals, much less pesticide runoff that can lead to fish kills and destroy habitats, and so on. Of course, they are also typically more expensive than conventionally grown produce.

So is organic worth it? We think so, because of the signifi-cant environmental benefits and the much lower toll on wildlife. From a health standpoint, though, the case is less ironclad.

Studies have shown that organic produce contains more antioxidants but on the whole does not have significantly more vitamins and minerals than conventional produce. And a study in the *British Journal of Nutrition* reveals that as many as 10 percent of organic fruits and vegetables have pesticide residue, a result of cross-contamination from nearby nonor-ganic farms. So *always* wash your fruits and vegetables, or-ganic or not!

If your main goal is healthy foods, don't worry if you can't always afford organic. As Dr. Michael Greger notes, "You re-ceive tremendous benefit from eating conventional fruits and vegetables that far outweighs whatever little bump in risk you may get from the pesticides." And the evidence is clear that the residue in fruits and vegetables is far less concentrated than the toxins in meat.

So, yes, if you want to make the right choice for the planet and its animal inhabitants, choose organic as much as possible. But you can safely feed your family conventional produce—just be sure to wash your fruits and vegetables thoroughly, and if you want to be more mindful, try to always go organic on the "dirty dozen," which are the more thin-skinned of the produce family (list courtesy of the Environ-mental Working Group):

continues

Should You Buy Organic Produce? *continued*

- Peaches
- Apples
- Sweet bell peppers
- Celery
- Nectarines
- Strawberries

- Cherries
- Pears
- Grapes
- Spinach
- Lettuce
- Potatoes

MISCELLANEOUS

Cooking aids. Extra-virgin olive oil, dark sesame oil, coconut oil, tomato sauce (always useful for last-minute meals), vegetable stock (low sodium), nutritional yeast (works wonderfully in bean sauces, soups, pasta, and on popcorn . . . it kind of makes things cheesy), whole-grain flour, arrowroot or cornstarch (for thickening soups, sauces, and stews), blackstrap molasses (just two tablespoons contains 400 mg of calcium—more than milk and cheese).

Condiments. Pick up salsa, soy sauce, vegetable bouillon, Sriracha sauce, vinegar, spicy peanut sauce, and nondairy salad dressing.

Spices. One of the silliest myths out there is that plant-based food is bland. Well, bland food is bland food, whether it's a chicken breast, steak, or tofu stir-fry. A few pinches of herbs and spices can turn your ho-hum plate into a mouthwatering symphony of tastes. Must-have herbs and spices include basil, garlic, ginger, oregano, cumin, turmeric, thyme, chili powder, red pepper, cinnamon, paprika, and curry powder.

And, most of all, make your list. Keep a basic one on your phone that you can riff off of regularly. Think about your meals in advance and then plan accordingly. As long as you plan your meals around protein, carbohydrates, and vegetables, you'll find that shopping becomes a quick and easy ritual. If you're prepared with a shopping list, you'll strut through those aisles with poise and purpose, and you'll return home a conquering hero ready for your week!

CHAPTER 12

How to Entertain, Pack a Lunch, and Feed Your Family

While some people can read an informative health or environmental book or see an undercover factory farm investigation and instantly give up animal food for life, others require a longer journey. If you want to move away from animal products, don't feel like you need to switch to clean protein all at once. The same is true for getting your family to join you. It's best not to traumatize the kids by tossing out all the old food and implementing your new clean protein regime while they're at school or while your significant other is at work. Sit down with your family and let them know that you'd like to start occasionally replacing meat with clean protein. Invite them to be part of the inquiry and shift.

Start small. Substitute the occasional veggie burger, then try buying almond or soy milk instead of dairy milk. You could swap out the cold cuts for clean protein alternatives. Or you might even try surprising the kids once in a while: look at the expression on your family's face when you inform them that they've been enjoying Earth Balance instead of butter or nondairy spread instead of cream cheese. (They likely will not have tasted the difference.) Be insistent that your family incorporate clean protein into their diet, and talk to them about why it's important to you; but don't be tyrannical about it. Introduce clean protein as an experiment, beginning with occasional meals and later progressing to days and then weeks at a time. Remember, every step away from animal protein is positive, and there's a great chance they will feel it rather quickly in their energy levels and body mass indexes.

By now you're likely pretty clear on the health benefits of clean protein, and you've seen how easy it is to shop for and cook with it. A few of your friends and maybe even your immediate family are interested, if not yet sold on it. So far, so good, right?

Now imagine this scene: It's time for your annual Super Bowl party, or you have to wine and dine a dozen guests. Your friends and family used to love your famous prime rib, that decadent crab bisque, that buttery Alfredo sauce. Imagine the look on their faces when you mention to them, "I'm not doing animal protein now, guys; I'm eating clean!" While your open-minded friends may be fine with it, others might grumble. Meanwhile, what if you're having trouble packing a quick, tasty lunch to bring to the office? Or there's someone holding out in your family, someone not as enthusiastic about clean protein as you are? What if everyone seems nervous that they're going to have to live on boring salads, never to enjoy their favorite fare again? Trust us; we want more than just salads, too. Way more. We have big appetites, love substantial plates of food, and want to feel as satisfied and nourished as anyone. But as you've seen and will continue to see in the recipe section, we really enjoy an abundance of hearty food and never feel lacking in taste, texture, or fulfillment.

———————

Not everyone you know is going to read this book and gain an in-depth understanding of clean protein, so it's up to you to make the change as easy as possible for your friends and family. It means preparing quick, healthy, and delicious food suitable for everyone. Don't worry—it's not as daunting as it seems, and, again, lean in as you feel comfortable and ready. As we'll see in this chapter, there are many simple ways to smooth the protein transition. It'll mean a little bit of compromising and some patience at first, but you are doing a wonderful service for your friends and family.

The main thing to keep in mind is that you want to frame it as "crowding out, not cutting out." Crowd out the old animal stuff with clean, healthy protein. That way you're not just getting rid of stuff that you're going to miss but rather adding in things that are nutrient packed and super satisfying. If you start out depriving yourself, this transition won't work. Instead, use this time as one of exploration: experiment with curiosity and excitement, positioning yourself as a foodie with a new mission. It's a mind-set!

HOW TO ENTERTAIN

The truth is that animal-based protein, while destructive to our health and environment, is habit. It's reliable. It's easy to prepare. So how do you entertain a house full of hungry guests clamoring for their old favorites?

The easiest way is to, well, stick to their old favorites . . . with a twist. When you're entertaining people who are not used to eating plant-based fare, it's a good idea to make your food look as familiar as possible. Your best friends Steve and Jackie are used to a big sausage and cheese pizza, then give them sausage and cheese pizza! Pizza dough is plant based, of course, and so is the tomato sauce, and you can buy both the crust and the sauce at any grocery store. If you want to get creative on your own, try sautéing veggie toppings in olive oil, like mushrooms, onions, and peppers. We love the meat alternatives like veggie sausage and pepperoni that you can find in many grocery stores and any health food store. (True, they aren't the most healthy things in the world, but they're so much cleaner than the animal-based products. And hey, it's the Super Bowl!) You can make your own clean protein "Parmesan" cheese by blending up some cashews with nutritional yeast and a pinch of salt—there are a ton of recipes on the web—or you can opt for one of the many nondairy cheeses you can find at the grocery store. Steve and Jackie don't just get their favorite pizza; they get a chance to see and taste just how good plant-based alternatives can be.

Fran wants her chicken wings? Try the Gardein or Beyond Meat's Beyond Chicken Strips—you just pop them in the toaster oven—and use whatever BBQ sauce or glaze you'd like. If you live in a big city that has a Chinatown nearby, you'll find some fantastic "mock wings" that are stunningly delicious, all made from grains and legumes. You can also find them online, through Amazon or Thrive Foods. If you want to be healthy about it, you can prepare your own clean protein wings with tahini, wheat gluten, and nutritional yeast. (We opt for simplicity, though, and get the frozen stuff!)

Anthony wants your famous chili? Give the man what he wants—but make it with black beans and some veggie meat crumbles. Karen wants a burger and her kids want hot dogs? There are so many great animal-free burgers and dogs in the freezer section of your favorite grocery store, and they're amazingly good. And really, it's all about the fixins and presentation. If you used to have cheeseburgers with pickles, tomatoes, mayo, and ketchup, do the same thing but just opt for the nondairy cheese and mayo with whatever brand of veggie burger is your favorite.

Dave can't do without his mac and cheese? No problem! Any macaroni will do, and you can use Daiya Cheezy Mac. And, again, you can also make your own plant-based cheese with nutritional yeast, but that might not taste as rich for your friends who want familiarity. A note here that bears repeating: you don't have to do everything so that it's ideally healthy and nutritionally perfect. You are providing a bridge to the better, and those transitional meals will be much more successful if they're tasty and fulfilling, reminding your guests that nothing is lost in the transition to clean protein. Additionally, you're probably getting as much or more protein than you would have with the meat or cheese of yesteryear.

Buffets are wonderful because you can put out an array of dishes that your guests can choose from, making it more likely that they find new things as well as old favorites that they like. Do a nice mix of salads, using all kinds of veggies and quinoa and chunks of whatever clean proteins you like to "beef" up the texture. Eggplant parm made with plant-based cheese; chickpea cakes topped with arugula; fajitas stuffed with black beans, avocado, and salsa; peanut stew with butternut squash . . . you get the drift. Show how abundant clean protein is, and how deliciously fulfilling it can be. Your guests will likely be surprised at how many options there are, and the food will likely spark a lively conversation about the future of protein.

Remember, for most people, the first step toward clean protein is realizing, "Hey! This is delicious!" Then comes, "Gawd, I feel so good on this stuff. . . . " But we digress.

The key is to prove to your skeptical guests that you can throw a fantastic dinner party using all clean protein, without making the food look like something out of the '70s hippie era. Plant-based food has come a long, long way since then. (Although we nod to that generation for their awareness and advances!) Rice and beans are great . . . but you can do better. That goes for you, too, pasta primavera. Remember, variety is the spice of life! If you're throwing a party, most of your guests aren't going to be planted in their chairs. They'll be talking and mingling and roaming your home, so include lots of decadent finger food. Think nondairy "mozzarella" sticks, sweet potato bruschetta, stuffed mushrooms, baked jalapeno poppers, and smoky avocado fries. There are also tons of things in the freezer section of Whole Foods, Trader Joe's, Costco, or whatever grocery store you're frequenting. Look for veggie dumplings, chickenless crispy tenders, meatless meatballs, and edamame.

As for entrees, remember that Americans are accustomed to protein at the center of the plate. Don't be afraid to offer your guests heaps of clean protein, whether it's sesame-crusted tofu, quinoa lentil loaf, or coconut-crusted seitan. Truth be told, though, you're more likely to impress with Beyond Meat's Beyond Burger, fishless filets from Gardein, pasta with Lightlife Smart Ground meat crumbles, Tofurky deli slices, or Field Roast sausage and peppers. Make it interesting, make it delicious, make it abundant.

Another fun idea is to try a theme. Barbeques are a great time to break out the veggie burgers and veggie dogs and put the grill to good use. You may have read that grilled food is unhealthy, but this is only true for animal protein. When you look at a charred hamburger or hot dog, those blackened grill lines are actually carcinogenic compounds. When animal flesh comes into contact with high heat, a chemical reaction occurs between the amino acids in animal protein and the creatine in muscle tissue. The reaction produces heterocyclic amines, known as HCAs, which in 2005, the federal government added to its list of known carcinogens in humans, and many studies before and since have proven this connection.

However, grilling plant-based foods is safe. Creatine is not found in clean plant protein, thus cancer-causing HCAs are not produced. So you can fire up the grill and throw on some delicious veggie burgers or dogs, vegetable kabobs (make sure to load on the sweet onions, pineapples, and peppers), tofu, tempeh—and perhaps most delicious of all, juicy portabella mushrooms. You can even use many of your favorite marinades that you once used on steaks, such as soy sauce, olive oil, lemon juice, Worcestershire sauce (use a clean blend that does not include anchovies), garlic, and pepper. Kathy's favorite is good ole A-1!

If you think your guests might balk at dishes built around meat alternatives, consider an Indian or Thai theme, which are both delicious, quick, and perfect for buffets. The best part is that so many staple Indian and Thai dishes are already plant based. Some Indian recipes call for using ghee, a form of clarified butter, but you can usually replace it with vegetable oil. As long as you steer clear of yogurt, cream, and paneer cheese recipes, you can easily veganize many dishes if they aren't already. (There are wonderful nondairy plain yogurts available in supermarkets these days, so check them out and add them into your recipes!) Try some vegetable samosas with chickpeas or vegetable pakoras as appetizers, then move on to lentil dahl and chana masala for mains. As for Thai food, replace meat with tofu, any fish sauce with soy sauce, and you can make your favorite curry or pad Thai. Your guest will have an incredibly satisfying meal without thinking twice whether there was animal protein involved! As long as someone is well fed and satisfied, the origin of the protein won't matter.

In all honesty, we often take the easy road and order out from a favorite Thai restaurant and ask for the green and red curry with tofu sans fish sauce, along with some rice and veggies. If the restaurant is run by Thai people, they have the spice combo down from generations of successful meals, and it's easier on busy days to just pour all that goodness into some serving bowls, heat it up, and serve on a festive table.

Final tip: never skimp on desserts. That is, if you want to have happy guests. And here's a little gift: chocolate is plant based. (Just make sure to avoid low-quality milk chocolate and look for 70 percent or higher content of cocoa.) Try a mousse made of almond or soy milk, cocoa powder, dates, and avocado all blended up in a food processor—it's decadent and sweet and chock full of protein to boot, so the protein, fiber, and healthy fat slow down the release of glucose from the dates. You can impress your guests with a rich clean protein "cheesecake" using tofu and cashews finished off with coconut cream, deep-dish apple pie with cashew cream drizzled atop, or peanut butter chocolate chip soy or almond ice cream—all dishes that are sweet but have some protein in them, too, if you opt for nut-based dishes.

What if you are attending someone else's dinner party? This can be trickier. Many restaurants offer plant-based dishes, and as a paying customer you can ask that they get creative (or go somewhere else). But no one wants to be that guy or gal who shows up at a friendly dinner party and complains to the hosts about the food. (Oh please don't do that!)

Here's what you do: call up your hosts and tell them that you don't eat animal stuff and you just wanted to let them know so that they don't waste a piece of chicken or steak on you. Be polite and gracious, offering to bring a dish or two so they don't have to worry about making you something special. (Bring extra; clean protein, animal-free dishes tend to be big hits, so be prepared to share!) Odds are, they'll have something for you anyway, but just don't expect it. Remember, this is not a time to pontificate about clean protein. You are an ambassador for clean eating, and you need to present yourself—and this way of eating—as easy, approachable, and fun. Be informative if people ask you questions, but be accepting of their choices.

HOW TO PACK YOUR LUNCH FOR WORK

If you work in an office, you might be thinking it's too time intensive to pack your own lunch every day. Sure, you can prepare it the night before, but with dinner, the kids, *Game of Thrones,* catching up on e-mails . . . it's easy to let it slip until the morning. And if you wake up late, forget about throwing a lunch together; you're just trying to get out the door on time. The problem is, though, that if you don't really plan lunch, you'll have to limit yourself to more expensive, less healthy takeout. One good option is to regularly make extra food at dinnertime so you have leftovers. Double or even triple the recipe, and immediately put the extra in containers for the next couple days, and if there's enough, store a few helpings in the freezer in labeled containers. If you're out at a restaurant, take a full half of it to go before you even start eating; the servings are usually too big and caloric anyway, so this routine could save your waistline and stretch your dollar. Keep a good stash of microwave-safe containers in your kitchen, and, presto, you have a system in place! Some foods taste even better the next day, such as soups and chili. In the summer months, we like big, chunky salads filled with clean proteins like chickpeas, marinated tofu, or meat alternatives along with an abundance of colorful veggies. If you keep your favorite salad dressing and sauce (we like spicy peanut, creamy vegan salad dressings, Sriracha, or, believe it or not, steak sauce) in the office fridge, you can make pretty much anything taste great.

But what if you want to mix it up? Sometimes it's a fun endeavor to take time and prepare a fresh lunch that you haven't had in a while—it gives you something to look forward to before your lunch break. But, unless you're a genuine morning person, when you're bleary-eyed after waking up, the last thing you want to do is spend forty-five minutes preparing an intricate lunch. The good news is that with a little bit of advance planning, you can pack a killer lunch in under five minutes.

At the beginning of the week, cook several cups of brown rice or quinoa and immediately refrigerate in a sealed container. (Rice cookers, which are inexpensive, are wonderful because they're hassle-free and always make a perfectly cooked grain.) These grains are the base of many lunches and will last you all week. While you're at it, roast up your sweet potatoes and any other vegetable that takes a little time to prepare, then seal them up tight in your fridge. For you OCD types (guilty!), you can have the ingredients for each day's lunch labeled and ready to go before the weekend is over.

One of the quickest lunch options is a grain bowl. Before you leave for work, prepare your rice or quinoa, toss in a handful of your favorite (cooked) beans (fine to use canned if you didn't have time to make them on the stove), some chopped raw vegetables, and whatever spices or seasoning you like. Toss it in the microwave at work for ninety seconds, and you're set. The clean protein and fiber will do wonders for your energy throughout the day.

For sandwich lovers, you can't go wrong with vegetables and hummus. Simply spread some hummus on whole wheat bread and drop on your favorite vegetables, such as tomato, lettuce, carrots, onion, and pickles. For extra credit, layer on some seasoned tofu or veggie bacon for protein. Alternatively, ditch the bread and wrap up your creation with a whole-wheat or corn tortilla. Toss in some peppers, beans, lettuce, cilantro, and as much clean protein as you can squeeze in.

Salads are a staple, of course, but you can get bored of the same old greens every day. Diversify! On Monday you can pack a tabbouleh quinoa salad with cucumber and avocado; on Wednesday you can mix it up with a Mexican tempeh salad with brown rice, spinach, and black beans; and you can end your healthy week with a bowl of kale and tofu, cilantro, sweet potato chunks, roasted broccoli, and tomatoes. You can also chop up a cooked veggie burger—they go great with salads and make them more of a hearty meal.

When your office mates are heading for the midafternoon do-nuts and cookies, you'll be amazed at how little you desire those sweets, because your blood sugar will be steady and your belly will feel satiated.

FEEDING YOUR FAMILY

There's a lot of hysteria on the Internet about how much protein growing kids need. Unfortunately, lots of parents believe that kids need to be loaded with animal protein to ensure they grow to their full potential. But again, as the science points out, the opposite is true. Children who are raised on plant-based diets tend to be healthier than kids raised on dairy and meat and experience less obesity, and are just as tall.

In fact, Dr. Michael Greger of nutritionfacts.org points to a 2010 study from the *American Journal of Clinical Nutrition* that concludes that by young adulthood, plant-based kids are "taller than their omnivorous classmates: 2.5 and 2.0 cm taller for boys and girls, respectively."

While kids who regularly eat animal protein aren't taller, they are heavier: over the past thirty years, the number of children who are considered overweight has more than doubled. Dr. Greger explains, "Once an obese child reaches age six, it's likely they'll stay that way. And even if they don't, being overweight in our youth predicts adult disease and death regardless of adult body weight, even if we lose it." And as the Physicians Committee for Responsible Medicine notes, "Adolescents raised on a vegetarian diet often find they have an easy time maintaining a healthy weight and have fewer problems with acne, allergies, and gastrointestinal problems than their meat-eating peers."

Studies have shown that an animal protein–rich diet can cause fatty streaks in the arteries of children as young as ten—the precursor to heart disease. So, it's imperative that our kids eat clean protein from as early an age as possible. PCRM publishes an excellent guide on their website (www.pcrm.org) for feeding kids of all ages. Once babies stop breastfeeding, an iron-fortified cereal is helpful to keep their iron stores high, followed by mashed fruits and vegetables by age one. Supplemented cereal is a common recommendation because it's easy on the baby's stomach and reliable. (By the way, this advice is exactly the same whether you follow an animal- or plant-based diet, advises Susan Levin, director of nutrition at PCRM—"an infant at about 6 months needs a reliable iron source in the diet—breast milk has some absorbable iron, but probably not enough for infants at this stage." Again, this is the advice for all babies.) At the six-month mark, experts recommend starting babies on solid foods, some of which should be good sources of iron.

Iron-fortified cereals specifically made for infants, especially rice-based ones, are recommended as first foods because they are hypoallergenic. But you don't have to do this. You could simply feed them good whole food sources, like mashed lentils, pureed beets, or blended spinach.

You can also introduce well-cooked clean proteins like tofu and beans around this age. (As always, be sure to design a baby's meal plan in consultation with medical professionals. But do choose a doctor or nutritionist who is up on the latest science regarding plant-based diets; if he or she doesn't seem supportive of your move away from animal foods, look for one who is.)

As for toddlers and young children, many parents become anxious with growth charts and runny noses. Moms and dads might be tempted to include animal protein to make sure everything is "normal," but your kids will easily thrive on a plant-based diet by following some basic tips. First, make sure they get enough calories in the form of high-fat plants. That might mean more than three meals per day, with an emphasis on calorie density. Think fewer grains (they can fill a child up before he or she takes in enough calories) and more high-fat nuts, avocados, and nut butters. In fact, as much as 50 percent of a young child's calories should come from healthy nonsaturated fats. Other ideas include protein- and healthy fat–rich tofu, full-fat nut milk, and plenty of smoothies. Pro tip on kid smoothies: add lots of frozen blueberries, as that will turn the smoothie a pleasing purple, which picky kids tend to love; it will also disguise whatever green you might have slipped into the liquid meal or snack! And remember to ensure that your child's foods are fortified with vitamin B12.

Kids and teenagers have busy schedules and high energy needs. And let's face it—school cafeterias tend to be nutritionally desolate places. At a time when public schools enter partnerships with Coca-Cola, Domino's, Pizza Hut, and other fast food restaurants, finding clean protein in a school can be nearly impossible. The few veggie options your school offers are likely processed and mundane, and kids will easily get bored. If your child's school does not offer quality plant-based options, you should speak up and petition the school. Bring it up at PTA and school board meetings, and get other parents to do the same.

But this can take time, and your kids' diets should not suffer while you wait for your school to take action. Consider packing your kids' lunches so you always know they are getting sufficient nutrition. You can also make sure they don't get bored with the same old cardboard veggie burger every day—oftentimes the only nod schools will give to nonanimal protein. To keep up with your kid's busy lifestyle, PCRM recommends ten daily servings of whole grains for teens aged thirteen to nineteen, one to two servings of dark green vegetables, three servings of other vegetables, four servings of fruit, and three servings of high-protein legumes, nuts, or nondairy milk.

Yes, this is a lot of food, and it means you have to plan accordingly. The good news is that your kids will love food that comes in big portions. For breakfast that could mean a bagel with hummus or peanut butter, and for lunch a big fat burrito with rice, beans, guacamole, salsa, and stuffed with your kids' favorite veggies. Or how about chickpea salad with a dab of vegan mayo and some whole grain crisp bread? A hearty bowl of mac and veggie cheese? A tofu-egg salad sandwich on sprouted bread? For snacks, consider dried fruit, veggies, and hummus dip, granola bars, trail mix, and lots of fruit. (You might take a gander at Kathy's book, *The Book of Veganish*, which is aimed at young adults and teens; there are a ton of teen-tested recipes and snack ideas therein!)

If you're having a tough time convincing your kids to move to clean, plant-based protein, try making their favorite dishes but with nonanimal versions of the ingredients. For meals that traditionally require eggs, such as pancakes and waffles, replace them with ground flaxseed. The general rule of thumb is to replace one egg with one tablespoon of ground flaxseeds and three tablespoons of water, although you can find conversion charts online to suit your individual needs; just search "plant-based egg substitutes" for products and charts. (In addition to being an excellent binding agent, flaxseeds have been proven to reduce your cancer risk and lower your blood pressure among countless other health benefits. They will also keep your kids, ahem, regular!) If you're baking cookies, cake, or other sweet pastries, applesauce and bananas are excellent substitutes for eggs and added sugars—and they make your creations decadently sweet, and, God forbid, healthy! Try substituting one to two mashed bananas for each cup of sugar in your recipe. Show your kids that nondairy ice cream is just as good as regular ice cream. It's important they understand comfort food can still be 100 percent plant based.

As with any shift in lifestyle, there will be good days and bad days, and there will be pushback. That's okay; just keep leaning into it. You can slowly phase out eggs, then chicken (there are so, so many wonderful chicken alternatives in the grocery freezer, so try them all to see which ones your family likes best), and so on. Or you can try meat-free days, starting with Meatless Mondays and building from there. There is no need to change all at once; in fact, it's more likely to be a fun and joyful experience that will take root if you're relaxed about it. Get excited and steer clear of dogma. There will be slipups and frustrations, and that's perfectly fine. Remember that you are providing an invaluable shift to your family: the gift of good health and soaring energy. You are making the environment cleaner, and your carbon footprint smaller. You are making the world a better, cleaner place, one serving of clean protein at a time.

Frequently Asked Questions

We know this might be a big shift for you, and you may still have questions about health and nutrition. So we've gathered the most common concerns and asked Dr. Neal Barnard, founder of the Physicians Committee for Responsible Medicine, to answer them for you.

Can too much plant protein be toxic?

It is really not possible to overconsume plant protein by eating vegetables, beans, grains, and fruits. These foods are so filling that, as we get the protein and other nutrients we need, our satiety cues are activated. In other words, we're full and we stop eating. Concentrated protein powders and bars are a different story. They can deliver unlimited protein, much more than the body needs, and they are not really necessary. That said, they do not appear to be harmful, so far as we can tell.

continues

Frequently Asked Questions *continued*

Can you get sufficient iron and calcium from clean protein?

First, we should be clear about what protein is. Sometimes we use the words "animal protein" as a synonym for "meat." But protein really is simply a long chain of amino acids, a bit like a microscopic string of beads, and it serves as building blocks for making various things in the body. Meat is muscle tissue, and it contains protein, fat, connective tissue, and occasional parasites from the animal it came from.

Meat does have iron. However, animals don't make the iron that is in their muscles. They simply ate plants that contained iron. And when we eat plants, we get iron in the same way. Greens and beans are loaded with it.

Meat is not a good source of calcium. While there is calcium in milk and other dairy products, cows do not actually make calcium. They merely eat the calcium that is in the vegetation they consume. When we eat plants, we get nature's original source of calcium. Greens and beans are great sources.

Animal products have lots of fat, whereas plant foods are leaner. Isn't fat good for us?

Remember that protein itself does not contain fat. Rather, muscle tissue (i.e., meat) has fat. And it has the wrong kind of fat. Animal products are very high in saturated fat, which the body does not need at all.

We don't require much fat in our diet; we need only small amounts of aptly named "essential" fats: alpha-linolenic acid (omega-3) and linoleic acid (omega-6). You'll get all of these essential fats in plants and in the recommended ratio (4:1, omega-6:omega-3).

continues

Frequently Asked Questions *continued*

Don't our bodies need some cholesterol to be healthy, and plant protein doesn't have any. Do I need to supplement?

We need only traces of cholesterol, and our bodies make all we need. We do not need any in our diets and are better off without it. Cholesterol is a bit like sticks of dynamite. It's very handy when you're trying to build a tunnel or dig a mine. But a little too much of it left in the wrong place, and you're in trouble. When we ingest dietary cholesterol or—even worse— animal fat, our bodies end up with far more cholesterol than we need. That leads to heart disease and may also increase Alzheimer's risk.

If I switch to animal-free protein, do I need to count the grams I consume to make sure I'm getting enough?

No. Protein is a natural component of vegetables, beans, grains, and fruits. As long as you are getting enough calories, you will get enough protein. And if you are an athlete, you'll naturally eat more food, and protein comes along with it.

Protein is a bit like oxygen. Oxygen is in the air, and when you breathe, you get the oxygen you need without thinking about it. And when you are physically active, you're breathing faster, so your body takes in more oxygen. So, if we eat foods from plant sources, we get protein. The more active we are, the more we eat, and the more protein we consume. There is no need for animal protein and no need for concentrated protein of any kind (e.g., protein powders). Your body sorted this out a long time ago; we just have to let it work.

continues

Frequently Asked Questions *continued*

Do I need to take care as I get older to get more protein? Is protein harder for my body to absorb as I age?

Some people have suggested that we need fewer calories and use protein less efficiently as we age. It is not clear that this is true for most people. But you can certainly favor beans and soy products, if you like. You'll easily get plenty of protein, without any need for animal products.

CHAPTER 13

How to Cook—Recipes!

Now's the fun part—making delicious meals using clean protein! You may or may not be a recipe person, but these are some of our favorites in case you want to follow along exactly or just glance at them for ideas of what you can try. What you're likely to find is that the potential for making hearty and fulfilling dishes is endless. Seriously, wasn't the routine getting old, cooking all that chicken or fish along with a side of vegetables? Once you've done some exploring and really dipped into this wonderful food, we think you'll look back on the old days of animal food as boring.

In the following section of the book, we've given you a little bit of everything to get started. There are recipes from traditional cultures all around the world, so that you can see that nonanimal protein has been around for a very long time. The reason it's been around so long is that the local people who have passed down and perfected the recipes have learned how to flavor very simple foods so that they taste sensational. Sometimes it's a matter of the right herbs and spices, and sometimes it's just getting the textures to be mouthwateringly pleasing.

We've also tapped some of the meat alternative companies we like so they could share what they've found their customers love.

Of course you can do pretty much anything with plant-based meats that you could with animal-based meats, but because they've tested so many recipes to see which ones get the best feedback, we're sharing those so you can branch out a little bit. A note here: if there is a recipe you like but you can't find that particular brand of "chick'n" or "sausage" in your grocery store, do any or all of the following: (1) call or e-mail the company to find out where their product is carried near you; (2) make a request to the store manager to order the product; they respond to customer desires and want to keep up with current trends; or (3) substitute another similar brand; they're all pretty darn good!

Lastly, some of our favorite chefs really know how to make clean protein taste unbelievably good; you might already be familiar with their culinary talents, but either way, you're in for a real treat with these recipes. If you like a particular chef's sensibilities more than the others, do go a step further and check out their own cookbooks to see more of their culinary magic! In any case, you'll have a robust mix of recipes, and we look forward to hearing from you about what you've tried and loved.

Get ready, get hungry; your life is about to change so deliciously!

BREAKFAST

Carob Peanut Butter Cup Smoothie Bowl Kid Friendly

By David Carter, the 300-Pound Vegan NFL defensive lineman

MAKES 2 SERVINGS (OR 1 IF YOU'RE A 300-POUND VEGAN)

This one might taste like a childhood favorite peanut butter cup, but it's more than 60 grams of protein in disguise. Sweetened naturally with bananas and dates, this is an ideal energy source for the serious athlete. Topping it off with crunchy peanuts, sesame seeds, and coconut turns this into an amazing textured chocolate frappe. Don't hold back—enjoy this smoothie bowl with abandon because it is just as nutritious as it is delicious!

Smoothie
½ cup hemp or other nondairy milk
4 bananas
2 tablespoons peanut butter
½ cup carob or cocoa powder
8 pitted dates

Toppings
1 banana, sliced thin
2 tablespoons unsweetened shredded coconut
¼ cup unsalted peanuts
2 tablespoons sesame seeds

Puree the smoothie ingredients until smooth. Pour into a bowl and top with any or all of the toppings.

First Kiss Smoothie

By Will Tucker, professional bodybuilder, fitness trainer, nutritionist

MAKES 1 SERVING

KF, BF: We thought this was an interesting recipe because it shows how the body can get amino acids from fruits without having to break down a long protein chain to get them.

Protein is made from chains of amino acids, which our bodies break down into human building blocks. While this recipe doesn't look like it contains protein on the surface, it contains all the essential amino acids we need, ready to be used to build muscle as is!

½ pink pitaya (dragonfruit) or ½ pack Pitaya Plus frozen pitaya
1 cup chopped mango
1 cup fresh strawberries, stems removed, ½ pound
Coconut water, to desired consistency, about 1½ to 2 cups
    (from young Thai coconut preferably)

Puree the ingredients together, pour, and enjoy.

NOTE: You can usually find frozen pitaya at Trader Joe's, Whole Foods, Walmart, and Target!

Sausage and Spinach Frittata

Recipe courtesy of Tofurky

MAKES 6 SERVINGS

This Tofurky Chick'n Apple Sausage and Follow Your Heart VeganEgg frittata is the answer to your brunch prayers. Fancy enough for company but simple enough for anytime, this dish will bring everyone together for a plant-based protein feast. Get creative and toss in some extra veggies—spice it up with hot sauce and a side of potato hash.

6 tablespoons Follow Your Heart VeganEgg powder
1½ cups ice-cold water
½ teaspoon salt
½ cup unsweetened coconut or soy creamer
1 tablespoon extra-virgin olive oil
2 packed cups baby spinach
⅓ cup chopped roasted red peppers
2 Tofurky Chick'n Apple Sausages, diced

Preheat the oven to 350°F.

In a medium bowl, whisk the VeganEgg powder with ice-cold water and salt until smooth, then whisk in the creamer.

In a medium oven-safe skillet, heat the oil to medium heat. Add the spinach and cook, stirring until wilted. Add the red peppers and sausage. Pour the egg mixture into the skillet, and stir until combined. Cook the mixture without stirring until it starts to pull away from the edges of the pan, about 5 to 7 minutes. Place the pan in the oven and cook until completely set, 15 to 18 minutes.

Southwest "Bacon" Breakfast Wrap

By Micah Risk, ultramarathoner, nutritionist, proud mama, and cofounder of Lighter Culture

MAKES 1 SERVING

Smoky, chewy bacon. Sweet, juicy tomato. Savory, rich avocado. Hearty black beans. Fresh, crispy spinach. All wrapped up in a simple tortilla for easy eating on the go.

4 slices Upton's seitan bacon
1 teaspoon olive oil
¼ avocado
1 flour tortilla
½ medium-size tomato, or
  1 Roma tomato, diced
¾ cup (about ½ can) cooked
  black beans, drained and rinsed
1½ cups fresh spinach
Salt to taste
Freshly ground black pepper
  to taste

Over medium heat, cook the seitan bacon in the olive oil for 2 minutes per side. Remove from the pan and allow it to cool until comfortable to handle. Chop the bacon into bite-size pieces. Scoop out the avocado and spread it on the tortilla. Spread the chopped seitan bacon and the remaining ingredients on the tortilla, wrap up, and enjoy!

Easy Oats in a Jar

By Jason Wyrick, cooking teacher, caterer,
former diabetic, executive chef of the Vegan Taste

MAKES 1 SERVING

I hate making breakfast. The easier it is, the better, but I still want something full of flavor that will keep me going for a few hours. Enter Easy Oats in a Jar. The rolled oats will soak up the yogurt and soften without cooking and turning mushy. The cherries lend a pop of sweetness, and the Brazil nuts give it a nice crunch. I also love bright flavors and heat, so I usually add the chile and lime. It's not for everyone, but if you love bold flavors, you'll love those options. Once you're done, seal it up in a jar for a delicious, transportable breakfast.

¾ cup rolled oats, uncooked
1 small container (5.5 ounces) nondairy yogurt
4 to 5 dried cherries
4 to 5 Brazil nuts, chopped
1 chile de arbol, optional
Zest of 1 lime, optional

Toss all the ingredients together, transfer to a jar, and let sit for at least 20 minutes.

NOTE: You can find chiles de arbol—little dried red chile peppers—in Hispanic markets, Whole Foods, and many other grocery stores. You can also order them online!

Red Lentil Flour Waffles with Smoked Almonds Kid ☀ Friendly

By Jason Wyrick, our new best friend,
whose food we're crazy for

MAKES 4 LARGE WAFFLES

Lentil flours, made from ground dried lentils, have been used to make crisp flatbreads throughout Asia for centuries. They also happen to make for a great, high-protein waffle batter. Couple that with chopped smoked almonds, bananas, and maple syrup, and you have a clean protein powerhouse that's great for your body, great for the planet, and great for your palate!

Waffles
½ cup red lentil flour (see Note)
½ cup whole wheat pastry flour or
   whole wheat flour
¼ teaspoon baking soda
½ teaspoon sea salt
1½ tablespoons granulated sugar
2 tablespoons applesauce
1 tablespoon canola oil or melted
   nondairy butter
1¼ cups almond milk
Juice of ½ small lemon
Oil

Toppings
Maple syrup
Pinch of salt
1 small banana, peeled and sliced
⅓ cup smoked almonds
   (use toasted slivered almonds if
   you can't find smoked almonds)

Whisk together the lentil flour, whole wheat flour, baking soda, sea salt, and sugar in a mixing bowl. Whisk into the dry mix the applesauce, oil or nondairy butter, almond milk, and lemon juice. Let this sit for 3 to 5 minutes while you heat your waffle iron. Brush or spray oil onto the waffle iron, and add ⅓ to ½ cup of the batter, depending on the size of your waffle iron. Close and cook for 5 minutes. Repeat until you are out of batter.

Combine the maple syrup with a pinch of salt and smother the waffles with it. Top with sliced bananas and smoked almonds.

NOTE: To make red lentil flour, grind 1¼ cups dried red lentils in a high-speed blender until completely powdered.

Gallo Pinto

Recipe by Jason Wyrick

MAKES 4 SERVINGS

Gallo pinto is the national breakfast, some might even say the national dish, of Costa Rica. It's made in the morning and served throughout the day. It's an easy dish of onions, peppers, rice, and beans, served with Salsa Lizano, a peppery hot sauce reminiscent of Worcestershire sauce found everywhere in the country. Although you can order Salsa Lizano online, feel free to substitute your favorite hot sauce. I had gallo pinto for breakfast every morning during my travels in Costa Rica, and this dish powered me through mornings of hiking, kayaking, zip lining, and just chilling out.

1 small onion, chopped
1 red bell pepper, stem and seeds removed, chopped
1 teaspoon olive oil
3 garlic cloves, minced
1 cup cooked long grain rice
1½ cups (14-ounce can) black beans, with liquid
½ teaspoon salt
½ teaspoon freshly ground black pepper
¼ cup loosely packed chopped cilantro
Salsa Lizano, or your favorite hot sauce
1 avocado, chopped

In a medium-size pot, sauté the onion and red pepper in the olive oil over medium heat until the onion just starts to brown, about 8 to 10 minutes. Add the garlic and cook 1 more minute. Add the cooked rice, beans, salt, and pepper, and cook for 3 to 5 minutes, until the rice has absorbed the bean liquid. Remove from the heat and immediately stir in the cilantro. Serve with Salsa Lizano and avocado.

SALADS

Black Bean Avocado Salad

Recipe by Jason Wyrick, executive chef of the Vegan Taste

MAKES 1 SERVING

This is one of the first salad recipes I created many years back when I cut dairy out of my diet, and it's still one of my go-tos. It's basically nachos on a plate with a healthy dose of avocado instead of cheese, and it's loaded with protein from the black beans. It's a toss-everything-in-a-bowl-and-eat-right-away salad, but if you want to kick it up a bit, you can take Mark Bittman's Tofu "Chorizo" recipe (page 206) and add half a cup warm for a satisfying southwestern bowl.

3 cups baby arugula or chopped lettuce, loosely packed
1½ cups (14-ounce can) cooked black beans, drained and rinsed
1½ cups baked blue corn chips
½ cup good-quality salsa
1 large avocado, chopped
¼ cup toasted salted pepitas (also known as hulled green pumpkin seeds)

Combine all the ingredients and serve immediately.

Roasted Eggplant and Artichoke Salad

Recipe by Jason Wyrick

MAKES 3 SERVINGS

This salad is a protein plate in disguise. Artichokes come in at just over 30 percent protein, highlighting how protein dense plants can be, while the chickpeas and eggplant are no slouches, either. Nutrition aside, though, this is an easy-to-make salad that's a meal, and I absolutely love the flavor of oven-browned artichokes and eggplant.

1 eggplant, chopped into bite-size pieces
2 cups artichoke hearts, 6 ounces
½ cup cooked, rinsed chickpeas
1½ tablespoons olive oil
1 teaspoon sea salt, divided
¾ teaspoon freshly ground black pepper
2 teaspoons fresh thyme leaves
¼ cup tahini
Juice of 2 lemons
¾ teaspoon Aleppo chili flakes or red chili flakes, optional

NOTE: Aleppo chili flakes have a medium heat with caramel notes and can be purchased online and at many spice stores. If you can't find Aleppo chili flakes, substitute a like amount of red chili flakes.

Instead of blending the tahini, lemon juice, and water you can use ½ cup of the Preserved Lemon Tahini Vinaigrette in the Plant Bowl recipe (page 166).

Preheat the oven to 450°F.

Toss the eggplant, artichokes, and chickpeas in the olive oil, then add ½ teaspoon of the sea salt, the pepper, and the thyme and toss again. Transfer to a baking dish, and roast for 15 minutes. Remove the dish from the oven, stir, and bake again for 10 more minutes. Set aside.

Blend the tahini, lemon juice, remaining ½ teaspoon of the salt, and 3 tablespoons water, pour over the salad, and toss. Dress with Aleppo chili flakes or red chili flakes, if you like.

Thai Beefless Mushroom Salad

Recipe by Jason Wyrick

MAKES 2 SERVINGS

This version of the classic Thai beef salad uses seared portabella mushrooms, fresh mint, and a salty and sweet sauce to create a refreshing salad as a meal. Although it's not traditional, you can add peanuts for some extra protein and crunch.

Mushrooms

2 medium-size portabellas, stems removed and sliced into ½-inch-thick strips
1 tablespoon sesame oil
¼ teaspoon salt
¾ teaspoon freshly ground black pepper
4 Szechuan peppercorns, ground, optional

Dressing

Juice of 3 limes
1 teaspoon of grated palm sugar or fine ground turbinado sugar
Pinch of salt
2 tablespoons vegetarian "oyster" sauce, or 2 tablespoons soy sauce

Salad

3 small shallots, thinly sliced
6 cherry tomatoes, halved
2 Thai long chiles, or 2 serrano chiles, minced
4 green onions, sliced
½ cup chopped cilantro, packed
2 tablespoons chopped fresh mint, packed
¼ cup roasted salted peanuts, optional
1 cucumber, peeled, halved lengthwise, and sliced

Over medium-high heat, sauté the mushrooms in the oil until they are browned, about 6 to 7 minutes. Toss them in the salt, pepper, and Szechuan peppercorns, if using.

Whisk together the ingredients for the dressing.

Toss all the salad ingredients together, reserving the cucumber, with the mushrooms and dressing. Serve and arrange the cucumber slices around the sides of the plates.

NOTE: Szechuan peppercorns have a numbing quality and slightly sour taste. If you don't have them, simply omit them.

Vegetarian "oyster" sauce can be found at most Asian stores and is typically made from shiitake mushrooms. It serves a similar purpose as fish sauce.

Thai long chiles are similar in flavor and heat to large serrano chiles.

Quinoa and Chickpea Tabbouleh Salad
(excerpted from *The Vegiterranean Diet*)

By Julieanna Hever, MS, RD, CPT, a.k.a. the Plant-Based Dietitian

MAKES 4 SERVINGS

Light and herb infused, this salad is refreshing and extremely nutritious. Traditionally made with bulgur wheat, this gluten-free version boasts similar flavors, but it's friendly for those eschewing gluten and more substantial because of the added chickpeas.

Zest and juice from one lemon
½ teaspoon freshly ground black pepper
½ teaspoon salt, optional
1 garlic clove, minced, optional
2 cups cooked quinoa, cooked according to basic instructions on package
1 (15-ounce) can chickpeas, rinsed and drained
1 large unpeeled cucumber, seeded and diced
¾ cup halved grape or cherry tomatoes
¾ cup finely chopped Italian flat-leaf parsley, packed
¾ cup finely chopped fresh mint leaves, packed
¼ cup finely chopped green onions

In a medium bowl, whisk together the lemon juice, lemon zest, pepper, salt, and garlic, if using. Fold in the quinoa, chickpeas, cucumber, tomatoes, parsley, mint, and green onions until thoroughly combined. Garnish with extra chopped herbs, if you like.

Fall Harvest Salad

Recipe courtesy of Daiya

MAKES 2 SERVINGS

KF: I will not lie; I was a cheese addict. No matter how much I realized that cow's cheese was detrimental to my health, I craved it and had a hard time giving it up. But then along came Daiya, and now I'm a happy (nondairy) cheese addict!

1 small acorn, butternut, or other hard fall squash
1 tablespoon olive oil for brushing
¼ cup chopped pecans
1 block Daiya smoked gouda, chopped
4 cups baby spinach leaves, loosely packed
¼ cup dried cherries
1 Honeycrisp apple, cored and chopped
½ cup cooked quinoa

Preheat the oven to 350°F.

Cut the squash in half, remove the seeds, and lightly brush with oil. Place cut-side down on a baking sheet, and roast until the squash is soft but not mushy, about 30 minutes. Peel and chop the squash into bite-size pieces. Set aside ½ cup of the squash for this salad. The remaining squash can be stored and used for other recipes.

Toast the pecans over medium heat in a skillet for 1 minute.

Combine all the salad ingredients and serve.

Fish-Friendly Tuna Salad Kid Friendly

By Colleen Patrick-Goudreau, cookbook author, speaker, podcaster

MAKES 4½ CUPS, ABOUT 3 SERVINGS

I grew up on tuna salad sandwiches; from childhood through young adulthood, they were one of my go-to lunches—until I stopped eating the critters of the sea. This version has a similar texture and the same satisfying fat content while leaving the animals alone.

2 cups raw sunflower seeds, soaked for at least 2 hours and up to 24 hours
2 garlic cloves, peeled
8 green onions, chopped (about ¼ cup)
½ red onion, diced
2 stalks celery, diced
2 carrots, diced
2 kosher dill pickles, diced
3 tablespoons diced parsley, packed
½ cup roughly chopped walnuts
1 tablespoon Dijon mustard
¼ cup eggless mayonnaise
½ to 1 teaspoon salt
Freshly ground pepper to taste

NOTE: Because the seeds need to soak for anywhere from 2 hours to 24, you'll want to factor that into your start-to-finish timing for this salad.

Drain and rinse the sunflower seeds. Add the sunflower seeds and garlic to a food processor, and pulse until the seeds are a textured paste. Scrape the sides with spatula, as needed, so you don't have large chunks of sunflower seeds. Transfer to a large bowl, add the green onions, red onion, celery, carrots, pickles, parsley, walnuts, mustard, mayonnaise, salt, and pepper to the bowl, and stir to thoroughly combine. Taste, and adjust seasoning as desired.

BOWLS

Broccoli Almond Miso Bowl

Recipe by Jason Wyrick, executive chef of the Vegan Taste

MAKES 2 SERVINGS

Calorie for calorie, broccoli has a higher percentage of protein than meat, a shocking fact for those of us raised in cultures where meat is considered the only viable protein. Now combine broccoli with miso, itself a protein heavyweight, along with rice and almonds, and you've got a healthy, satisfying, umami-strong meal all in one bowl. This is the epitome of plant strong.

¼ cup white miso, or miso of your choice
¼ cup orange juice
2 cups broccoli florets, steamed
1 cup cooked short-grain brown rice
¼ cup toasted slivered almonds
1 teaspoon shichimi (a Japanese seven-spice chili blend), optional

Whisk together the miso and orange juice. Toss with the broccoli. Add the rice to the bowls, then add the broccoli and sauce, followed by the almonds. Sprinkle generously with the shichimi, if using.

Plant Bowl

By Matthew Kenney, restaurateur, star chef

MAKES 4 SERVINGS

KF: To eat at one of Matthew Kenney's restaurants is to dine in haute style and experience his culinary genius. Although this recipe is not for someone in a hurry, I highly recommend trying it when you have a little time. . . . It's beyond delicious.

1 small kabocha squash, peeled, seeds removed

3½ tablespoons olive oil, divided

1½ teaspoons sea salt, divided

1½ cups sprouted quinoa (see note)

2 cups sprouted black lentils (see note)

6 leaves lacinato kale, chopped into large bite-size pieces

½ cup Piquillo Romesco (see recipe below)

Preserved Lemon Tahini Vinaigrette (see recipe below)

1 large avocado, sliced

Pea shoots for garnish, optional

Preserved Lemon Tahini Vinaigrette

½ cup tahini

⅓ cup cold water

2½ tablespoons lemon juice

1 preserved lemon skin

¼ teaspoon sea salt

Piquillo Romesco

2 cups piquillo chiles from a jar, chopped

1 cup almonds, toasted

½ cup olive oil

¾ teaspoon smoked paprika

¼ cup sherry vinegar

1 Fresno chile, seeds removed

½ serrano chile, seeds removed

1 garlic clove

1 teaspoon sea salt

NOTE: To sprout lentils: Rinse and drain well. Transfer the lentils to a bowl and cover them with 2 inches of water. Let them sit for 12 hours. Drain, rinse the lentils, and drain again. Transfer to a jar and secure with a sprouting lid or cheesecloth. Turn the jar upside down at an angle so the liquid can drain and air can circulate through the jar. Keep the lentils at room temperature and out of direct sunlight. Rinse and drain the lentils twice a day until they sprout. Once they do, drain them and keep them refrigerated for use.

To sprout quinoa: follow the directions for sprouting lentils, but your initial soak time is 6 hours instead of 12 hours.

Preheat the oven to 400°F.

Cut the kabocha squash into 2-inch-long, ½-inch-thick pieces. Steam them for 5 minutes. Transfer to a baking dish and toss them in 2 tablespoons of the olive oil and ½ teaspoon of the sea salt. Roast the squash for 30 minutes. Remove from the heat and set aside.

While the squash is roasting, bring 1¾ cups of water to a simmer in a small pot, add the quinoa, and bring back to a simmer. Cover the pot and cook for 10 minutes. Drain, if necessary, and set aside.

Over medium heat, sauté the sprouted, uncooked lentils in 2 teaspoons of olive oil with a pinch of salt for 3 to 5 minutes. Transfer to a bowl and set aside.

Over medium heat, sauté the kale in 2 teaspoons of olive oil and a pinch of salt until the kale leaves turn a vibrant color, about 2 to 3 minutes. Transfer to a bowl and set aside.

To make the vinaigrette, purée all the Preserved Lemon Tahini Vinaigrette ingredients until smooth. Repeat with the Piquillo Romesco ingredients to make the romesco sauce.

To assemble the bowls, smear the romesco sauce around the side of the bowls. Place the quinoa in one half of the bowl and the lentils in the other half of the bowl, as best you can. Drizzle the vinaigrette on top, then place 3 or 4 pieces of squash in each bowl, 3 or 4 slices of avocado in each bowl, and 3 or 4 pieces of kale in each bowl. Garnish with pea shoots if you like.

NOTE: Kabocha squash is a type of Japanese winter squash similar to pumpkin, but with a green skin. These can be found at most Asian markets, Whole Foods, and similar stores.

Lacinato kale, also known as dinosaur kale and Tuscan kale, has long, dark, narrow leaves with a sweeter, more delicate flavor than curly kale.

Preserved lemons are lemon skins that have been pickled in a brine of lemon juice and salt, popular in North African cuisine. You can most easily find these at markets specializing in Middle Eastern ingredients.

Mongolian BBQ Seitan Bowl   Kid Friendly

By Chloe Coscarelli, founder of ByChloe restaurant chain, star chef

MAKES 4 SERVINGS

Once, when we photographed this dish, half of the photo team ditched their ordered-in lunches for a bowl of Mongolian BBQ Seitan. This dish is sticky, savory, and sweet, and almost effortless to make.

¼ cup hoisin sauce
1 tablespoon soy sauce
1 tablespoon agave
1 teaspoon lemon juice
1 to 2 teaspoons chile garlic sauce
2 tablespoons canola oil
8 ounces shiitake mushrooms, stemmed and sliced
8 ounces seitan, cut into thin strips
2 teaspoons grated fresh ginger

⅛ teaspoon ground cinnamon
⅛ teaspoon ground cloves
4 ounces snow peas, strings removed
2 green onions, trimmed and thinly sliced
¼ cup chopped fresh cilantro, packed
2 cups cooked rice, for serving

To make the sauce, whisk together the hoisin sauce, ¼ cup water, soy sauce, agave, lemon juice, and chile garlic sauce in a small bowl and set aside.

In a large skillet, heat the oil over medium-high heat and stir-fry the mushrooms and seitan until lightly browned and the mushrooms have released their juices, about 2 to 3 minutes. Add the ginger, cinnamon, and cloves and stir-fry 2 more minutes.

Add the sauce and snow peas to the skillet. Reduce the heat to medium and cook until the sauce has thickened. This may happen quickly. Turn off the heat and mix in the green onions and cilantro. Serve over rice.

Peanutty Perfection Noodle Bowl Kid Friendly

By Chloe Coscarelli

MAKES 4 TO 6 SERVINGS

This is my favorite recipe in the book. Super creamy, slightly sweet, and subtly spicy—noodle nirvana.

1 cup coconut milk
¼ cup maple syrup
¼ cup soy sauce
½ cup peanut butter, chunky
    or creamy
1 tablespoon chile garlic sauce
1 teaspoon grated fresh ginger
3 garlic cloves, minced
2 tablespoons lime juice
1 tablespoon toasted sesame oil

1 pound brown rice (or other
    whole grain) noodles
3 green onions, trimmed and
    thinly sliced
2 carrots, peeled and shredded
½ cup peanuts, roughly chopped,
    for garnish
2 tablespoons roughly chopped
    fresh cilantro, packed, for
    garnish

To make the sauce, combine the coconut milk, ½ cup water, maple syrup, soy sauce, peanut butter, chile garlic sauce, ginger, and garlic in a medium saucepan. Let the sauce cook over medium heat, whisking frequently, until it comes together and thickens, about 5 to 7 minutes. Remove from heat and whisk in the lime juice and sesame oil.

While the sauce is simmering, bring a large pot of heavily salted water to a boil. Add the noodles and cook according to the package directions. Drain, rinse with cold water, and briefly drain again.

Toss the hot noodles with the sauce, green onions, and carrots. Garnish with the peanuts and cilantro and serve. Any leftovers can be served warm or cold the next day for a delicious lunch.

HANDHELD EATS

Bean and Squash Tortillas with Papaya Salsa

By Dan Buettner, National Geographic explorer,
founder and author of *The Blue Zones* (and Kathy's boyfriend!)

MAKES 6 SERVINGS

Nicoyans are among the longest-living, healthiest people in the world. They eat tortillas at every meal, so the choice of when to eat this is all yours! For variety, substitute a mango or pineapple for the papaya in the salsa.

Papaya Salsa
1 small ripe papaya, peeled, halved, seeded, and diced, about 1 cup
1 small red bell pepper, stemmed, cored, and diced, about ½ cup
¼ cup diced fresh cilantro leaves, packed
3 tablespoons olive oil, divided
2 tablespoons fresh lime juice

Beans and Veggies

1½ cups cooked, rinsed black or pinto beans

1 medium yellow squash, chopped

1 cup corn kernels, preferably fresh

2 medium carrots, peeled and shredded

1 teaspoon ground cumin

Up to ½ teaspoon ground dried cayenne

¼ teaspoon salt

Tortillas

6 corn tortillas

Combine the papaya, bell pepper, cilantro, 1 tablespoon of the olive oil, and the lime juice in a small bowl. Cover and set aside at room temperature for up to 4 hours.

Heat 1 tablespoon of the oil in a large skillet over medium-high heat. Add the beans, squash, corn, carrots, cumin, cayenne, and salt. Cook, stirring often, until the squash is tender, about 5 minutes. Stir in the papaya salsa. remove from the heat, and set aside.

Heat the broiler. Lay the tortillas on a baking sheet and brush them with the remaining 1 tablespoon of oil. Broil until warmed and lightly toasted, about 30 seconds.

Transfer each tortilla to its own serving plate and top with the bean and salsa mixture.

Tacos and Sopes with Smashed Frijoles de Olla

Recipe by Jason Wyrick, executive chef of the Vegan Taste

MAKES 12 STREET TACOS OR 6 SOPES

Tacos and sopes, one fashioned from a thin tortilla, the other a thick boat of toasted masa, are transformed into culinary magic with the simple addition of beans and salsa. Add avocado and a few other garnishes, and you have heaven right in your hand. These traditional foods have fueled Central America for centuries, and they are as easy to make as they are to eat.

Your choice of either 12 street-size (4-inch-diameter)
     corn tortillas or 6 sopes
2 cups smashed Frijoles de Olla (page 205) or
     vegetarian refried beans, warmed
¾ cup salsa roja or your favorite salsa
2 avocados, chopped
¼ cup minced white onion, rinsed (see Note)
3 tablespoons minced cilantro, packed
Lime wedges, 6 for sopes, 12 for tacos
¼ cup toasted salted peanuts, optional
2 ancho chiles, diced and fried (see Note)

NOTE: Rinsing your minced onion removes much of the compound that causes onion to have a bite and cause tearing.

To fry the chiles, snip away the stem and shake out the seeds. Dice the chiles. Add enough oil to a small skillet to make a thin layer and bring it to medium heat. Add the chiles, slowly stir, and cook for about 30 seconds, then immediately remove them from the oil.

If using tortillas, warm a tortilla by laying it in a dry pan for 5 seconds, then flipping it and letting it sit for another 5 seconds. If using sopes, toast, flat-side down, for 30 seconds over medium heat, then flip and toast for another 20 seconds before filling.

Fill the tortillas or sopes with smashed beans, then salsa, then chopped avocado. Top with a sprinkle of minced onion and minced cilantro, and serve with lime wedges. You can also top them with peanuts for crunch and fried chiles for a shot of spicy caramelized chile flavor.

NOTE: Sopes are thick disks of corn about 4 inches in diameter with a raised lip that forms a boat into which you can load your ingredients. You can find premade sopes at most Mexican markets.

Black Bean Plantain Burrito with Pineapple Salsa

Recipe by Kayla Roche, courtesy of MUSE school (MUSE is the first fully plant-based, sustainable living school in the country)

MAKES 4 SERVINGS

Burritos are an all-time favorite at MUSE. This Caribbean-inspired burrito is great any time of the day, and the pineapple salsa is great to make whether or not you're in the mood for a burrito!

Pineapple Salsa
2 cups diced pineapple, preferably fresh
½ medium-size red onion, minced
¼ cup chopped cilantro, packed
Juice of 1 large lime
¼ teaspoon salt

Burrito Filling
2 tablespoons olive oil, divided
1 ripe plantain, sliced diagonally into ¼-inch-thick pieces
¾ teaspoon salt, divided
½ medium-size red onion, minced
½ red bell pepper, minced
2 garlic cloves, minced
¼ teaspoon chili powder
½ teaspoon ground cumin
2 cups cooked black beans, drained and rinsed

Tortillas and Finishing Ingredients
4 spelt or whole wheat tortillas
Pineapple Salsa
1 avocado, sliced
Hot sauce to taste, optional
Chopped cilantro for garnish

To make the salsa, combine all the salsa ingredients in a small bowl, cover, and chill. This will keep for up to 5 days refrigerated.

To make the burrito filling, heat 1 tablespoon of olive oil over medium-high heat in a medium-size skillet. Once the oil is hot, add the plantains and sprinkle with ¼ teaspoon of salt. Fry the plantains until they are well browned, about 2 to 3 minutes per side. Remove from the pan and set aside.

Return the pan to the medium-high heat, and add 1 tablespoon of olive oil. Add the onion and bell pepper, and cook until the onions just start to brown, about 3 to 4 minutes. Add the garlic, and cook 1 more minute. Add the chili powder, cumin, and ½ teaspoon of salt, stir for 30 seconds, then add the beans and give a quick stir. Remove from the heat and smash the beans a few times with the back of a large stirring spoon or potato masher, just enough to give them a rough texture.

Warm the tortillas by placing them individually in a dry pan set at medium heat for 5 to 10 seconds per side. Fill with the bean mix, then add the plantains and wrap them closed. Smother with pineapple salsa, then top with sliced avocado, followed by hot sauce, if using. Finish the burritos off with a sprinkle of cilantro.

Kid Friendly

Quick Idea!

Need something fast? You can make a cheesy bean burrito with three ingredients. Roll up some vegetarian refried beans and Daiya shredded cheese in a tortilla, toast it on each side for a minute or so, and you've got a delicious meal ready to go that you can also package up and take with you to work.

Sweet Potato Black Bean Burger

Kid Friendly

By David Carter, the 300-Pound Vegan,
all-around amazing athlete and human

MAKES 4 TO 6 SERVINGS

KF: When I first met David and his wife, Paige, I wondered how such gorgeous, super-successful people could be so down to earth, but once I realized that they're guided by their ethics, it became clear that kindness is everything to them. But by the way, check out the protein dose in this recipe!

Burger Patty

2 medium-size sweet potatoes,
    chopped into large pieces
1 cup rolled oats
1 cup cooked quinoa, cooked
    according to package directions
1½ cups (15-ounce can) black beans,
    drained and rinsed
1 small red onion, minced
½ cup chopped cilantro, packed
2 teaspoons ground cumin
1 teaspoon chili powder
1 teaspoon chipotle powder
½ teaspoon salt
1 tablespoon olive oil or sunflower oil

Buns and Toppings

4 to 6 whole wheat burger buns
Raw onion rings or grilled
    onion strips
Smashed avocado
Chopped Roma tomatoes
Grilled or sautéed sliced
    mushrooms

Preheat the oven to 400°F.

Line a baking sheet with foil and spread the sweet potato pieces on the foil. Roast the sweet potatoes for 30 to 40 minutes, until soft. Allow the sweet potato pieces to cool, then peel them. Mash them and set them aside. Pulse the oats in a food processor until they are coarsely ground but before they turn into oat flour.

In a large mixing bowl, mix together the mashed sweet potato, oats, quinoa, beans, onion, cilantro, spices, and salt. Gently press the mix together until it is combined into a burger "dough." Take 1 cup of the mixture and form it into a patty. Repeat until you are out of the mixture. Refrigerate for 30 to 60 minutes.

Add the oil to a large skillet and heat to medium. Add the patties and cook 5 to 10 minutes per side, until slightly crisped on the outside.

Toast the buns if you like, and serve with any or all of the toppings.

Range-Free Gooey St. Louie Burgers

Recipe courtesy of Hungry Planet, plant-based meat company

MAKES 4 SERVINGS

KF: The founders of this company, Todd Boyman and his sister Jody, are friends of mine who are highly motivated to feed people clean protein without using animals or harming the environment. The company is based in the Midwest; the burgers themselves are gluten-free, high in protein, and very low in calories. With zero cholesterol or saturated fat, this burger, served with an ice-cold beer (or a lemonade) along with some fries is pretty much perfection on a plate.

Cheesy Filling
¼ cup plant-based Cheddar
  cheese (like Daiya or Follow
  Your Heart)
2 tablespoons plant-based cream
  cheese (like Tofutti or Daiya)
1 teaspoon Dijon mustard
2 tablespoons minced fresh
  parsley, packed
2 green onions, thinly sliced

(Plant-Based) Meat Mixture
1 pound Range-Free "ground beef"
½ teaspoon paprika
½ teaspoon garlic powder
½ teaspoon onion powder
1 teaspoon salt
½ teaspoon black pepper

Buns and Toppings
4 hamburger buns
Butter lettuce, or lettuce of
  your choice
Sliced tomato
Sliced sweet pickles

In a small bowl, mix together the Cheddar cheese, cream cheese, mustard, parsley, and green onions.

In another bowl, thoroughly combine the Range-Free "ground beef" with the spices. Shape this mixture into eight equal patties. Spoon the cheese mixture onto the center of four of the patties, leaving at least a ½-inch space clear around the edge of the patties. Place the remaining four patties on top of the bottom patties and cheese mixture, and seal the bottom and top patties closed by pressing the edges together. You should end up with four thick patties in total, each with a cheese filling in the center.

Broil the burgers on the top rack of your oven for 4 to 5 minutes on each side, or grill or sauté them over medium-high heat, covered, for 4 to 5 minutes per side.

Toast the buns, if you like, and serve the burgers with any or all of the toppings.

Thanksgiving Tofurky Sandwich

Recipe courtesy of Tofurky

MAKES 2 SERVINGS

After a formal Thanksgiving dinner, nothing tastes quite as right as a messy, gooey grilled vegan cheese Thanksgiving sandwich. The good news is that you already did most of the work the day before.

¼ cup cranberry sauce, plus more
    for dipping
4 slices rye sandwich bread
4 slices Tofurky Roast or
    6 Tofurky Peppered Deli Slices
4 slices nondairy Swiss or
    provolone cheese
2 tablespoons nondairy butter,
    divided

Spread 2 tablespoons of the cranberry sauce on 2 slices of bread. Add Tofurky slices, then cheese slices, and then close the sandwiches.

In a medium skillet, melt 1 tablespoon of the butter over medium heat. Place a sandwich in the pan and fry until browned and crisp on the bottom, about 5 minutes, then flip and repeat. Remove the sandwich, add the remaining tablespoon of butter to the pan, and repeat with the second sandwich.

Lentil and Tempeh Sloppy Joes

By Katie Lee, Food Network superstar specializing
in southern cooking and beach cuisine

MAKES 4 SERVINGS

I do love my comfort foods, so I make healthier versions of my favorites. Growing up, I loved sloppy joe night! Now I make a guilt-free lentil and tempeh version that's amazing. I usually serve them with baked sweet potato fries.

Sloppy Joe Mix

1 tablespoon olive oil

1 medium-size onion, diced

1 green bell pepper, diced

3 garlic cloves, minced

8 ounces tempeh, pulsed in a food processor into large crumbles

1 (4-ounce) can chopped green chiles

1 tablespoon chili powder

1 cup cooked green or brown lentils

1 (8-ounce) can tomato sauce

½ cup organic ketchup

1 tablespoon dark brown sugar

1 tablespoon Dijon mustard

1 tablespoon anchovy-free Worcestershire sauce

2 teaspoons cider vinegar

½ teaspoon celery seed

½ teaspoon salt

½ teaspoon freshly ground black pepper

Buns and Toppings

4 whole wheat buns

Sliced avocado

Pickles

In a large skillet, heat the olive oil over medium heat. Add the onion and bell pepper and sauté until the onions are translucent and the bell pepper is tender, about 7 to 8 minutes. Add the garlic and cook about 1 more minute. Stir in the crumbled tempeh, chiles, and chili powder, and cook for 2 to 3 minutes, stirring occasionally. Stir in the lentils, tomato sauce, ½ cup water, ketchup, brown sugar, mustard, Worcestershire, vinegar, celery seed, salt, and pepper. Reduce the heat to low. Cover and simmer for 15 minutes.

Toast the buns, if you like, add the sloppy joe mix, then 3 to 4 pieces of sliced avocado per sandwich, and serve with pickles on the side.

Chicken of the Woods Mushroom Sandwiches

By Chad and Derek Sarno of Wicked Healthy

MAKES 2 SERVINGS

We believe that using mushrooms as meat is the future of plant-based food! This recipe will show you how to transform a chicken of the woods mushroom into something meaty and magical using our wicked awesome pressing technique. Serve these with our suggested toppings on a bun or with your favorite plant-based side dishes!

Mushrooms
3 to 4 tablespoons canola or
  grapeseed oil, divided
2 large (chicken-breast-sized)
  chicken of the woods mushrooms
1 tablespoon fresh thyme leaves,
  chopped, or ½ tablespoon dried
  thyme
¾ teaspoon poultry seasoning
¾ teaspoon garlic powder
½ teaspoon granulated onion
⅛ teaspoon sea salt
⅛ teaspoon freshly ground black
  pepper

Buns and Toppings
2 whole wheat buns
Non-dairy cheese of your choice
A few leaves chard or spinach
Shaved red onion
Nondairy chipotle mayo

Preheat the oven to 350°F.

Add 2 tablespoons of oil to a cast-iron or heavy-duty pan and heat to medium. Once the oil is hot, lay the mushrooms in the pan and place a heavy lid or weight on top of the mushrooms. Cook for 2 minutes and flip the mushrooms. Add half the dry spices to the top, then return the weight. Cook for 2 more minutes, flip, season, and add the weight again. Continue cooking and flipping the mushrooms until they are lightly golden brown and no liquid remains in the pan. Remove from the heat.

Transfer the mushrooms to a sheet pan and roast for 10 minutes. Top with the nondairy cheese, and roast for 5 more minutes.

Lightly steam the buns for a few seconds, if you like, then toast them in the oven or in the cooking skillet so they can absorb the residual flavors in the pan. Add the mushrooms to the buns and use any or all of the toppings.

NOTE: You can get chicken of the woods mushrooms at Whole Foods, some higher-end markets, and markets that specialize in mushrooms.

Cornmeal Crusted Chick Seitan

Recipe courtesy of Upton's Naturals

MAKES 4 SERVINGS

Oil of your choice for brushing
⅓ cup nondairy milk
1 tablespoon cornstarch
½ cup cornmeal
2 tablespoons nutritional yeast or nondairy Parmesan
1 teaspoon garlic powder
1 teaspoon dried parsley
¼ teaspoon salt
1 pound (2 packages) Upton's Naturals Chick Seitan,
    broken into bite-size pieces

Heat the oven to 375°F.

Line a baking sheet with foil or parchment paper and lightly brush with oil.

In a small bowl, whisk together the nondairy milk and cornstarch. In a separate bowl, whisk together the cornmeal, nutritional yeast or nondairy Parmesan, garlic powder, parsley, and salt.

Dip the seitan pieces into the nondairy milk mixture, then dredge through the cornmeal mixture until thoroughly coated. Transfer to the baking sheet, and bake for 15 minutes. Flip the pieces, and bake 15 more minutes.

Serve with marinara or your favorite dipping sauce.

Avocado Beyond Chicken Sushi Roll

Recipe courtesy of Beyond Meat

MAKES 2 ROLLS

½ cup cooked sushi rice or other short-grain rice
2 sheets nori
6 to 8 Beyond Meat Beyond Chicken Strips
1 avocado, sliced
1 medium-size cucumber, peeled and cut lengthwise
    into ¼-inch-thick strips
Tamari or liquid coconut aminos
Pickled ginger

Spread the rice on the sheets of nori, leaving a 1-inch-wide uncovered space on one side of each sheet of nori. Layer the Beyond Meat Beyond Chicken Strips, sliced avocado, and cucumber over the rice on the end opposite the uncovered side. Lightly wet the uncovered section of nori. Starting with the side covered with the filling, roll the nori closed as tightly as possible, then press the wettened section of nori down onto the roll to seal it. Eat as is, or wet a sharp knife and cut into sushi medallions. Serve with a side of tamari or liquid coconut aminos and pickled ginger.

Take-with Protein Bar

Recipe by Jason Wyrick

MAKES 8 BARS

When I'm heading out to do a long hike or bike ride or when I'm going to be gone from the house for hours at a time, I like to take one or two of these high-protein bars with me. They're highly portable, hearty, and satisfying, and two of these are packed with enough energy to sustain me throughout the day. Once you make the bars, wrap them in plastic wrap, and you can store them in your fridge for up to two weeks.

¼ cup almonds (smoked almonds for an extra flavor boost)
¼ cup roasted salted peanuts
¼ cup toasted salted pepitas
¼ cup toasted sesame seeds
Salt to taste
Chipotle chili flakes to taste, optional
¼ cup unsweetened shredded coconut, toasted
12 pitted dates
Zest of 2 oranges

Pulse the almonds and peanuts in a food processor two or three times, until very roughly chopped. Toss the nuts, pepitas, sesame seeds, salt, chipotle flakes (if using), and shredded coconut together. Grind the dates together in a food processor and smash them into a paste, along with the orange zest. In a mixing bowl, thoroughly incorporate the nut mix into the date mix. Form into 8 bars.

You can eat them as is, or lay them on a baking sheet lined with parchment paper and dehydrate them at your oven's lowest setting for 6 to 8 hours, flipping them halfway through the cook time.

SOUPS AND STEWS

Ikarian Stew

By Dan Buettner, Mr. Blue Zones

MAKES 4 SERVINGS

KF: I often tell Dan I'd be with him just for this stew; it's that good.

This is hands-down my favorite longevity recipe. The savory one-pot meal fuses the iconic flavors of Ikaria, Greece, with the faintest hint of sweet fennel. As is customary in Ikaria, a small amount of olive oil is used to sauté the vegetables, then a generous drizzle finishes the dish. This practice is instinctively brilliant: heat breaks down the oil, so saving most for a final drizzle assures its rich flavor and maximum health benefits. This protein-rich stew freezes well, though the kale will lose a little of its vibrancy. To refresh the stew, add a few more fresh slivered leaves when reheating.

2 cups dried black-eyed peas

½ cup extra-virgin olive oil, divided

1 large yellow or white onion, diced (about 1½ cups)

1 medium fennel bulb, trimmed, halved, and sliced into thin strips

2 teaspoons minced garlic

3 large carrots, peeled and chopped (about 1 cup)

1 large red globe, beefsteak, or heirloom tomato, diced (about ¾ cup)

2 tablespoons tomato paste
2 bay leaves
1 teaspoon salt
4 large kale leaves, slivered
½ cup chopped fresh dill

Put the black-eyed peas in a large pot, add enough water to submerge them by 2 inches, and bring to a boil over high heat. Boil for 1 minute. Set aside off the heat and soak for 1 hour, then drain.

Warm ¼ cup of oil in a large pot or Dutch oven set over medium heat. Add the onion and fennel and cook, stirring often, until soft, about 8 minutes. Add the garlic and cook until fragrant, about 20 seconds. Stir in the black-eyed peas, carrots, tomato, tomato paste, bay leaves, and salt. Add just enough water to cover the ingredients in the pot, and stir vigorously until the tomato paste dissolves. Raise the heat to medium-high, and bring to a boil. Cover, reduce the heat to low, and simmer slowly until the black-eyed peas are tender but not mushy, about 50 minutes.

Stir in the kale leaves and dill. Cover and cook until the kale is tender, 5 to 10 minutes.

Discard the bay leaves. Ladle into four bowls. Drizzle 1 tablespoon of olive oil on top of each serving.

> *Tip:* For a quicker, no-fuss meal, substitute 4 cups of frozen black-eyed peas, thawed, or 4 cups of drained and rinsed canned black-eyed peas for the 2 cups of dried black-eyed peas. Simply add all the ingredients to the pot and simmer for 25 minutes, then serve.

> *Tip:* When working with high-acid foods like tomatoes or vinegar, always cook in nonreactive cookware, such as stainless steel, anodized aluminum, or enameled cast-iron pans, pots, and skillets.

Ash-e Anar—Pomegranate Split Pea Soup

By Jason Wyrick, executive chef of the Vegan Taste

MAKES 4 SERVINGS

Ash, pronounced *ahsh*, is simply a thick, herbal soup with a focus on legumes. These types of soups are such a foundational component of Persian cuisine that cooks are often called *ashpaz*, which translates to "maker of ash." They are delicious, warming, and rub-your-tummy satisfying. This particular one is made from yellow split peas and pomegranate molasses, an ingredient that transforms this dish from a simple split pea soup to one brought to life with a perfect balance of tart and sweet.

Soup

1 white onion, diced

3 tablespoons olive oil

4 garlic cloves, minced

1 teaspoon grated fresh turmeric or ½ teaspoon dried ground turmeric

½ teaspoon ground cinnamon

½ cup yellow split peas

½ cup rice (basmati works best)

1½ teaspoons salt

1½ cups chopped parsley, packed

1½ cups chopped cilantro, packed

½ cup chopped mint, packed

½ teaspoon freshly ground black pepper

¼ cup pomegranate molasses

Garnish

¼ cup olive oil

6 garlic cloves, sliced thin

2 tablespoons dried mint

¼ cup pomegranate seeds

Over medium heat in a 2- to 3-quart pot, sauté the onion in the oil until it turns translucent and just barely starts to brown, about 4 to 5 minutes. Add the garlic and sauté 1 more minute. Add the turmeric and cinnamon, quickly stir, then immediately add 6 cups of water. Add the split peas, rice, and salt. Cover, reduce the heat to low, and cook for 1 hour, until the split peas and rice are falling apart. Add the parsley, cilantro, mint, pepper, and pomegranate molasses, stir, and cook 20 more minutes. Remove from the heat and salt to taste.

For the garnish, in a pan, bring the olive oil to medium heat and add the garlic. Sauté the garlic until it browns, about 2 to 3 minutes. Remove from the heat and immediately add the dried mint to the oil to make a garlic, mint, olive oil mix. Add the soup to the bowls, spoon the oil mix onto the top of the soup, and sprinkle a few pomegranate seeds on top.

NOTE: Pomegranate molasses is a thick, sweet astringent syrup made from pomegranate juice and can be found at stores that specialize in Middle Eastern cuisine.

Sopa de Habas—Fava Bean Soup
(excerpted from *Vegan Mexico**))

By Jason Wyrick

MAKES 3 TO 4 SERVINGS

This easy soup, traditionally served during Lent, is full of rich, deep caramelized flavors from sautéed onions, garlic, and tomatoes. The key is cooking everything down to make sure all the flavors are intensified. You can also make this with pinto beans instead of fava beans. Nopales, sliced cactus paddles from prickly pear cactus, make a frequent appearance in this soup, but if you don't have fresh nopales, simply omit them.

1 tablespoon olive oil
1 medium yellow onion, coarsely
    chopped
5 garlic cloves, coarsely chopped
4 Roma tomatoes

3½ cups cooked fava beans,
    divided
½ teaspoon ground cumin
¾ teaspoon salt
1 to 2 chipotles in adobo, minced
1 cup sliced nopales, optional

*Recipes from *Vegan Mexico* copyright © 2016 by Jason Wyrick. Used by permission, Vintage Heritage Press.

Heat the oil in a medium pot over medium heat. Add the onion and sauté until it is well caramelized, about 15 minutes. Add the garlic and sauté 2 more minutes. Add the tomatoes and cook until they are reduced, 7 to 8 minutes. Transfer the onion mixture to a blender, along with 1 cup of the fava beans, 2 cups of water, cumin, salt, and chipotles, and purée. Transfer the purée back to the pot, and add the remaining 2½ cups fava beans and nopales, if using. Simmer the soup for 8 to 10 minutes and serve.

Smoky White Bean Chowder
(excerpted from *The 30-Day Vegan Challenge*)

By Colleen Patrick-Goudreau

MAKES 4 SERVINGS

You will love the flavors and simplicity of this thick chowder, perfect for any day of the week, any season of the year.

1 tablespoon nondairy butter, olive oil, or water for sautéing

1 medium yellow or white onion, chopped

6 garlic cloves, minced

3 stalks celery, diced

3 medium carrots, peeled and diced

2 bay leaves

2½ cups vegetable stock, or 2½ cups water mixed with a veggie bouillon cube

2 large yellow waxy potatoes, like Yukon Gold, peeled and diced

1 cup plain soy creamer or ½ cup canned coconut milk mixed with ½ cup water

3 cups or 2 (15-ounce) cans navy, great northern, or cannellini beans, drained and rinsed

½ to 1 teaspoon liquid smoke

½ teaspoon smoked paprika or hot or sweet paprika

Red chili flakes, optional

Salt and black pepper, to taste

Extra stock or creamer, as needed

Parsley and shredded carrots, for garnish

Plant-based bacon for garnish, chopped, optional

Heat the butter, oil, or water in a large pot over medium heat. (KF: If you want to go oil-free, you could also sauté the veggies in a dry pot rather than with water.) Add the onion and garlic, and sauté until they are softened and slightly caramelized, about 4 minutes. Stir in the celery and carrots. Add the bay leaves, stock, and potatoes. Cover and simmer until the potatoes are soft, about 20 minutes. Stir the soup every 4 or 5 minutes.

Remove from the heat and mash using a potato masher, breaking up the potatoes a bit. Alternatively, you can use an immersion blender, but don't completely purée. The final soup should be thick and chunky.

Add the creamer, beans, liquid smoke, paprika, red chili flakes (if using), and salt and pepper. Return to the heat and simmer, uncovered, for another 15 minutes.

The finished soup should be chowder thickness. If it is too thin, simmer uncovered for 10 minutes more. If it is too thick, add a small amount of stock or creamer to thin it. Garnish with parsley, shredded carrots, and plant-based bacon, if using. Serve with Saltine crackers.

Khumbi Haleem—Pakistani Mushrooms and Daal with Naan

Recipe by Jason Wyrick

MAKES 4 SERVINGS

This stew is magic in a bowl. Not only is it loaded with healthy protein from the daal, mushrooms, and barley, it's absolutely packed with flavor. If you don't have access to the different daals used in this stew, you can easily make this with red lentils. This is a simplified version of the traditional Pakistani dish that uses curry powder instead of toasted whole spices, but for those of you who want to kick this up a level, toast and grind your own spices and use fresh turmeric in place of the curry powder.

¼ cup nondairy butter, divided
3 cups diced cremini mushrooms,
   about ¾ pound
1 large yellow onion, diced
6 garlic cloves, minced
2 tablespoons grated fresh ginger
½ cup channa daal + ½ cup urad
   daal + ½ cup mung daal, or
   1½ cups red lentils
½ cup barley

½ cup wheat berries soaked for
   1 hour, optional
3 tablespoons curry powder
1 tablespoon garam masala
Generous pinch saffron
1 teaspoon salt
8 cups baby spinach leaves
Naan for serving
Lemon wedges, chopped fresh
   cilantro, sliced jalapeno, and
   sliced ginger for garnish

In a 3- to 4-quart pot, heat 2 tablespoons of the nondairy butter to medium high. Add the mushrooms and cook until they are well browned, about 5 to 6 minutes. Remove them from the heat and set them aside. Add the remaining 2 tablespoons of nondairy butter and reduce the heat to medium. Add the onion and cook until it starts to brown, about 6 minutes. Add the garlic and ginger and cook 2 more minutes. Add the daals or red lentils, the barley, wheat berries (if using), 6 cups of water, spices, saffron, and salt. Stir and bring to a simmer. Cover the pot, reduce the heat to low, and cook for 40 minutes.

Remove the stew from the heat and rapidly beat the daal so it becomes creamy. Immediately stir in the spinach and mushrooms while the stew is hot. Ladle into bowls and serve with naan, or your favorite flatbread, and any or all of the garnishes.

Elevate it: Instead of curry powder, use 2 teaspoons of grated fresh turmeric and toast and grind the following spices: ½ teaspoon of fenugreek seeds, 3 tablespoons of coriander seeds, 1½ tablespoons of cumin seeds, and 6 dried red chiles.

Curried Red Lentils with Charred Spring Onions and Field Roast Smoked Apple Sage Sausage

Recipe Courtesy of Field Roast

MAKES 4 SERVINGS

KF: High-protein sausage without the cholesterol, saturated fat, or yuck factor of animal sausage; yes please!

1 medium-size yellow onion, diced
2 tablespoons olive oil
2 tablespoons yellow curry powder
1 tablespoon ground cumin
6 cups vegetable stock
2 cups red lentils
Salt to taste
1 large sweet potato, peeled and diced
Freshly ground black pepper to taste
4 to 6 spring onions
2 links Field Roast Smoked Apple Sage Sausage

In a 4- to 6-quart pot, sauté the onion in the oil over medium heat for 4 minutes. Add the curry powder and cumin and sauté for 2 more minutes. Add the stock, lentils, salt to taste, sweet potato, and black pepper, and bring to a low simmer. Simmer the soup for 20 to 25 minutes, until the red lentils are soft and starting to dissolve.

Light your grill and let it heat to a medium heat. Grill the spring onions until the outside is charred. Set aside. Grill the Field Roast sausages for 4 minutes, rotating them every minute. Rub away some of the charring on the spring onions and slice them into ½-inch-long pieces. Slice the Field Roast sausage into ¼-inch-thick medallions.

Ladle the soup into the serving bowls and top with the Field Roast sausage and charred spring onions.

SAVORY EATS

Wild Mushroom Tuscan White Bean Pizza Kid Friendly

Recipe by Jason Wyrick, executive chef of the Vegan Taste

MAKES 1 PIZZA, 2 SERVINGS

Travel to Italy, and you'll be constantly enticed by the heavenly aroma of olive wood–fired thin-crust pizzas. These pizzas focus on high-quality pizza dough made with a fine-grain flour and fresh, local ingredients. Often, these pizzas are devoid of animal products entirely, celebrating instead vegetable-forward deliciousness with a myriad of sauces, from simple olive oil and garlic, to a classic marinara, to thin bean spreads reminiscent of a good-quality hummus. This particular pizza uses a white bean dip popular throughout Tuscany, coupled with wild mushrooms, and crisped sage. Talk about clean protein!

½ cup dried wild mushrooms
1 cup hot water
¼ cup olive oil, divided
2 tablespoons chopped fresh sage
½ cup cooked cannellini beans, drained and rinsed
1 garlic clove
Juice of 1 medium-size lemon
½ teaspoon salt
Prepared pizza dough for 1 pizza crust, preferably
    made from type 00 flour for pizza

Heat the oven to the highest setting, typically 550°F, with a pizza stone in the center of the oven. If you don't have a pizza stone, line a sheet pan with foil and generously oil the foil.

Soak the wild mushrooms in the water for 10 minutes, then remove from the water and pat them dry. (Note that you can save that soaking water for a soup base or to use in other recipes.) In a medium-size skillet, heat 1 tablespoon of the oil to medium-high. Add the mushrooms and cook until lightly browned, about 2 minutes. Add the sage and cook 1 more minute, then remove from the heat.

Purée the remaining olive oil, beans, garlic, lemon juice, and salt until you have a thick spread.

Roll out the pizza dough, then smear the white bean spread all around it. Top with the mushrooms and sage. Transfer the pizza to the pizza stone and bake until the rim is crisp, about 3 to 4 minutes.

NOTE: Type 00 flour refers to a very fine grind on the flour, ideal for making the perfect pizza crust. When purchasing this type of flour, make sure you get the 00 flour for pizza, as there is also 00 flour for bread and these are not the same.

Pizza Marinara with Porcini Mushrooms and Truffle Cheese

Recipe by Jason Wyrick

MAKES 1 PIZZA, 2 SERVINGS

This pizza is more than it seems. You can use the same ingredients, minus the pizza crust, to make a great pasta sauce or even as a light soup. It's a riff on the classic pizza Napoletana using a soft almond cheese instead of mozzarella, and that soft almond cheese, comparable in protein to a dairy cheese, is completely devoid of cholesterol and high in flavor.

¼ cup dried porcini mushrooms, 2 ounces
1 cup hot water
2 tablespoons olive oil
4 garlic cloves, minced
1 (14-ounce) can San Marzano tomatoes, pureed
½ teaspoon salt
1 teaspoon fresh oregano, packed
Prepared pizza dough for 1 pizza crust, preferably made from type 00 flour
⅓ wheel Kite Hill Truffle, Dill, & Chive Cheese
3 to 4 shredded basil leaves

Heat the oven to the highest setting, typically 550°F, with a pizza stone in the center of the oven. If you don't have a pizza stone, line a sheet pan with foil and generously oil the foil.

Soak the porcini in the water for 10 minutes, then remove from the water and pat dry. (Note that you can save that soaking water for a soup base or for use in other recipes.) In a small pot, heat the olive oil to medium heat. Add the porcini and cook them until lightly browned, about 5 to 6 minutes. Remove the porcini from the pot, leaving as much olive oil as possible, and set them aside. Add the garlic to the pot and cook for 1 minute. Add the pureed tomatoes, salt, and oregano, and simmer for 5 minutes.

Roll out the pizza dough and spread ⅓ cup of the sauce on top. Top with the porcini and crumble the cheese on top. Transfer the pizza to the pizza stone and bake until the rim is crisp, about 3 to 4 minutes. Remove from the oven and immediately top with the shredded basil.

NOTE: Use a non-dairy mozzarella instead of the truffle cheese to make this kid-friendly.

Stuffed Acorn Squash

By Dan Buettner, from *The Blue Zones*

MAKES 8 SERVINGS

Ounce for ounce, quinoa packs a bigger protein punch than most whole grains do. Serve with a large green salad, and you have all your bases covered—fruit, vegetable, grain, fiber, greens, protein, and complex carbohydrates. If blood oranges aren't available in your area, use tangerines. They're not as pretty, but they're just as good.

4 large acorn squash (about 1 pound each), stemmed, halved, and seeded

1 tablespoon extra-virgin olive oil, plus more for the baking sheet

6 medium green onions, trimmed and thinly sliced

1 small celery stalk, diced (about 3 tablespoons)

½ cup dried cranberries, blueberries, currants, or raisins

½ cup chopped walnuts

⅓ cup dried apricots, soaked in warm water for 15 minutes, drained, and diced

1 teaspoon dried sage

2½ cups cooked long-grain brown rice, such as basmati

1½ cups cooked red or white quinoa

½ cup freshly squeezed blood orange juice

½ teaspoon salt, preferably sea salt

½ teaspoon freshly ground black pepper

Heat the oven to 350°F.

Lightly oil a baking sheet large enough to hold all the squash halves. Place the squash, cut-side down, on the prepared baking sheet, then transfer to the center of the oven. Bake until tender, about 30 to 40 minutes. Remove the squash from the oven, and leave them on the baking sheet. Let the squash cool for 5 minutes. A wire cooling rack on which to place the baking sheet works best here.

About 10 minutes before the squash is done baking, warm the oil in a large skillet over medium heat. Add the green onions and celery, and cook, stirring often, until the celery is softened but not browned, about 3 minutes. Add the dried berries, nuts, dried apricots, and sage. Cook, slowly stirring, until warmed through, about 2 minutes.

Add the rice, quinoa, blood orange juice, salt, and pepper. Continue cooking, stirring often, until hot, about 2 minutes. Remove from the heat and set aside. If your squash is not done cooling, cover the quinoa and rice mix to keep it warm.

Flip the squash over, and transfer to a platter or your dining plates. Stuff the quinoa and rice mixture into the squash to serve.

Bourguignon Stuffed Kuri Squash

By Deborah Pavain, executive chef and
proprietor of Gentle Gourmet Café

MAKES 6 SERVINGS

This has been a standing favorite at the restaurant. It is interesting because it is traditional with a serious plant-based and nutritional twist with the very colorful red kuri (Hokkaido) squash.

3 red kuri (Hokkaido) squash (use acorn squash if
    kuri squash is not available)
1 large onion, minced
2 large shallots, minced
2 tablespoons olive oil, divided
21 ounces seitan, cut into bite-size cubes

12 button mushrooms, quartered

2 bay leaves

1 sprig fresh rosemary, plus more for garnish

2½ liters (3 bottles) of good Bourgogne (Burgundy) wine

½ cup tomato purée

1 tablespoon prepared yellow mustard

¼ cup vegetable stock

Salt to taste

Pepper to taste

6 purple carrots, peeled and cut into bite-size cubes

2 teaspoons cane sugar, divided

4 large parsnips, peeled and cut into bite-size cubes

NOTE: If you don't have squash, you can serve this in a bread bowl, over a slice of toasted sourdough bread, over rice, or even just by itself.

Preheat the oven to 350°F.

Cut each squash in half, and scoop out the seeds and fibers. Line a baking sheet or dish with foil, and lightly oil it. Place the squash halves, cut-side down, and roast for 25 minutes.

While the squash is roasting, sauté the onions and shallots over medium heat in a 4-quart pot with 1 tablespoon of the olive oil until they are soft, about 5 minutes. Stir in the seitan, mushrooms, bay leaves, and one sprig of rosemary. Pour in the wine, tomato purée, mustard, and vegetable stock, and give a quick stir. Bring to a simmer for 45 minutes. Add salt and pepper to taste.

In a separate pan, sauté the carrots over medium heat with ½ tablespoon of olive oil until they are lightly browned, about 6 to 7 minutes. Add 1 teaspoon of sugar, shake the pan a couple of times, and cook 1 more minute. Add the carrots to the wine sauce. Add the parsnips and ½ tablespoon of olive oil to the pan and repeat.

Place each red kuri squash half on a plate, and fill with the bourguignon. Top each with a fresh sprig of rosemary, and serve.

Tuscan Fisherman's Soup—Cacciucco

By Gabriele Palloni, personal plant-based chef in Florence, Italy

MAKES 4 SERVINGS

The Livornese Cacciucco is a poor fisherman's soup, a typical dish from coast of Tuscany. My version uses pistachios in the shell instead of shellfish, urad daal to make the cakes instead of using ground fish, and wakame to add that oceanic flavor. The steps in this recipe can take awhile, but the time spent reducing the sauce and treating each component properly is well worth the effort.

1¼ cups urad daal
2-inch-piece wakame seaweed
½ cup pistachios in their shell
¼ cup sunflower oil
1 garlic clove, minced
3 tablespoons chopped Italian parsley, packed, divided
1 small red chile of your choice, minced
3 tablespoons extra virgin olive oil
Zest of 1 lemon
1 cup white wine
½ cup tomato sauce
2 cups vegetable stock
Salt and pepper to taste
4 slices Italian bread, toasted and sliced in half

Soak the urad daal in 4 to 6 cups of water with wakame seaweed for at least 4 hours. Drain, retaining the soaking water and wakame. In a separate bowl, soak the pistachios for 4 hours.

Dice the wakame. Whisk the urad daal and half of the rehydrated wakame to get a creamy mixture. If necessary add a little of the soaking water. Wet your hands and form disks about 1 inch thick and the size of your palm.

In a large skillet, heat the oil to just above a medium heat. Fry the urad daal disks until golden brown, about 3 minutes per side. Set aside on a paper towel to drain.

In a separate saucepan, sauté the garlic, 2 tablespoons of parsley, the chile, and the remaining wakame in the olive oil for 30 seconds, then add the lemon zest and stir quickly a couple times. Add the pistachios and white wine and cook until the wine evaporates. Remove the pistachios and keep them for a garnish, leaving behind bits of fried garlic, chili, wakame, and zest in the pan. Return the pan to the heat and add the tomato sauce and 3 tablespoons of the soaking water. Cook until the sauce becomes very thick. Add the vegetable stock, salt, and pepper, and cook at a boil for 10 minutes.

Place two halves of bread in each bowl, then smother with the soup. Top with the urad daal cakes, and garnish with the pistachios and minced parsley. Drizzle olive oil on top to finish each dish.

Seitan Jagerschnitzel
(excerpted from *Vegan Without Borders*)

By Robin Robertson, renowned cookbook author

MAKES 4 SERVINGS

Thinly sliced seitan absorbs the flavor of the rich mushroom sauce in these German "hunter's cutlets." You can use any kind of mushrooms you like, but I prefer using a variety to add interest and flavor dimension to the dish.

2 tablespoons olive oil, divided

4 seitan cutlets or 8 ounces seitan, thinly sliced

Salt to taste

Freshly ground black pepper to taste

1 small yellow onion or 2 shallots, minced

1 teaspoon tomato paste

8 ounces fresh mushrooms (single variety or assorted), thinly sliced

⅓ cup dry white wine

1 tablespoon soy sauce

½ to 1 teaspoon caraway seeds, crushed or whole

1 teaspoon sweet Hungarian
    paprika
½ teaspoon dried thyme, optional
1½ cups vegetable stock

1 tablespoon cornstarch dissolved
    in 2 tablespoons water
½ cup vegan sour cream

Heat 1 tablespoon of the oil in a large skillet over medium heat. Add the seitan, and season to taste with salt and pepper. Cook until browned on both sides, about 5 minutes. Remove the seitan from the skillet, and set aside on a plate. Cover with aluminum foil to keep warm.

Return the skillet to the heat and add the remaining tablespoon of oil. Add the onion and sauté until softened, about 5 minutes. Add the tomato paste, mushrooms, wine, soy sauce, caraway seeds, paprika, and thyme, if using. Cook, stirring frequently, for about 3 minutes.

Add the stock, and bring to a boil. Stir in the cornstarch mixture, decrease the heat to a low simmer, and cook, stirring constantly, until the sauce has thickened and the mushrooms are tender, 2 to 3 minutes. Stir in the sour cream. Taste and adjust the seasonings, if needed. Return the seitan to the skillet and continue to cook until the seitan is heated through, 1 to 2 minutes.

Hot Fried Maitake Chick'n

By Derek and Chad Sarno of Wicked Healthy

MAKES 2 TO 4 SERVINGS

Delicious, fun, and finger-licking good! Here's our wicked healthy take on southern fried chicken that uses whole chicken of the woods (maitake) mushroom clusters and shows that eating plants has never been easier or sexier. Shake and bake!

1 pound whole chicken of the woods mushroom clusters
Olive oil for brushing the mushroom clusters
1 tablespoon poultry seasoning
½ cup of your favorite hot sauce
3 cups all-purpose flour

1 tablespoon coarse grind sea salt

1 tablespoon finely ground black pepper

3 cups Follow Your Heart VeganEgg wash mixture (see package directions)

3 cups panko bread crumbs

3 cups crumbled kettle-cooked BBQ potato chips

1 cup canola or grapeseed oil for frying

Heat a cast-iron skillet or heavy duty saucepan over medium heat.

On a large baking sheet, lay out the mushrooms and lightly dab oil onto them, just enough so that the seasoning will stick to them. Sprinkle ¼ of the poultry seasoning onto the top of the mushrooms, then transfer to the skillet, seasoned-side down. Place a weight on top of the mushrooms, like a heavy lid, to create a press. Cook for 2 to 3 minutes, then flip over and season again. Repeat until all the seasoning is used and the mushrooms are lightly golden brown, with no liquid remaining in the pan. Remove from the heat and allow the mushrooms to cool.

In a bowl, toss the mushrooms in hot sauce, cover, and allow them to marinate for at least 1 hour, or overnight.

Set up a breading station with three separate bowls. In the first bowl, combine the flour, salt, and pepper. In the second bowl, add the VeganEgg mixture. For the third bowl, pulse the panko bread crumbs and potato chips in a food processor until coarse, then transfer to the bowl.

Add ¼ to ½ inch of oil to a cast-iron frying pan and heat to medium. Once hot, take a chicken of the woods mushroom cluster and dredge it through the flour, then the VeganEgg mix, and finally into the bread crumb and potato chip mix. Transfer to the oil and fry until golden brown, about 3 to 5 minutes. Transfer to a paper towel to drain. Repeat with the remaining mushrooms and serve.

NOTE: You can make these ahead of time and reheat them in the oven at 350°F for 5 to 10 minutes.

Spaghetti Squash Meatless Meatballs   Kid ☼ Friendly

Recipe courtesy of Gardein

MAKES 4 SERVINGS

KF: This is one of my favorites because I feel like I'm getting my veggies in (spaghetti squash!) while also indulging in comfort food (meatballs!). It's great for family dinners because kids and adults love it!

Spaghetti Squash
1 small spaghetti squash, split in half lengthwise and seeded
Olive oil for brushing
¼ teaspoon salt
¼ teaspoon freshly ground black pepper

Gardein Meatballs
1 package Gardein meatballs (8 meatballs)
1 tablespoon olive oil

Marinara
3 tablespoons olive oil
10 shallots or 1 medium-size white onion, diced
2 garlic cloves, thinly sliced
1 (28-ounce) can San Marzano tomatoes
1 sprig thyme, or 1 teaspoon fresh thyme leaves
¾ teaspoon salt
½ teaspoon freshly ground black pepper

Finishing Ingredients
2 tablespoons nondairy butter or olive oil
¼ cup loosely packed thinly sliced basil leaves
2 tablespoons Follow Your Heart Parmesan

> **Time-saving tip:** Make the meatballs, then the marinara sauce just after the squash goes into the oven.

To make the squash, preheat the oven to 450°F.

Rub olive oil along the inside of both halves of the squash, and dress with salt and pepper. Line a baking sheet with aluminum foil, and place the squash halves, cut-side down, on the sheet. Roast for 30 to 40 minutes, until you can stick a fork through the squash. Remove the squash from the oven, and allow it to cool until you can comfortably handle it. Using a fork, scrape the strands of squash from the skin and toss them with salt and pepper.

To make the meatballs, bring 1 tablespoon of olive oil to medium heat in a medium-size skillet. Add the meatballs and fry them, shaking the pan every minute or so, until they are browned, about 5 to 7 minutes. Remove the meatballs from the pan and set aside.

In the same pan, add 3 tablespoons of olive oil, and bring it to a medium heat. Add the shallots or onion and garlic, and cook until lightly caramelized, about 5 minutes. Add the tomatoes and juice in the can and the thyme, bring to a simmer, and reduce the heat to low. Simmer the sauce for 30 to 40 minutes, smashing up the tomatoes using a potato masher, whisk, or other sturdy utensil. Add the salt and pepper, and stir. Add the meatballs to the sauce, and stir a couple times.

Once your spaghetti squash is ready, toss it with 2 tablespoons of nondairy butter or olive oil, and transfer to the serving plates or a big platter. Smother with the meatballs and sauce and garnish with sliced basil and Follow Your Heart Parmesan.

Smoky Sweet Potato Boats   Kid Friendly

By Jenny Bradley for Miyoko's Kitchen

MAKES 2 SERVINGS

KF: Sweet potatoes + cheese + black beans = delicious protein heaven. Order Miyoko's cheese online if you can't find it in the grocery store!

2 medium-size sweet potatoes, pierced with a fork and wrapped with foil
1 shallot, minced
3 garlic cloves, minced
2 teaspoons olive oil
1½ cups (1 can) cooked black beans, drained and rinsed

3 cups loosely packed spinach
Salt and pepper to taste
1 cup unsweetened soy milk
½ wheel (3¼ ounces) Miyoko's Creamery Aged English Smoked
    Farmhouse nondairy cheese
Nondairy sour cream for garnish
Sliced avocado for garnish
Chopped green onions or chives for garnish

Preheat the oven to 400°F.

Place the sweet potatoes on a baking sheet and roast them until they are soft, 40 to 50 minutes. Reduce the heat to 350°F and remove the sweet potatoes from the oven. Unwrap them and cut them in half lengthwise. Scoop out the inside, leaving enough sweet potato intact to make sturdy sweet potato boats. Return these to the oven, cut-side down, unwrapped, and bake for 10 more minutes, then set aside.

While they are baking, sauté the shallot and garlic with the olive oil over medium heat in a medium-size skillet just until the shallots are soft, about 2 minutes. Add the black beans and warm through. Add the spinach, stir, and cook 1 more minute. Add salt and pepper to taste, and set aside.

In a small pot, heat the soy milk over medium heat, and add the ½ wheel of cheese. Whisk together until the cheese has melted.

Fill the sweet potato boats with the black bean and spinach mixture, and pour the cheese sauce on top. Top with any or all of the garnishes.

Gigantes Plaki—Greek Beans in Tomato Sauce

By Kiki Vagianos, publisher of thegreekvegan.com

MAKES 8 SERVINGS

There's a reason that certain places in Greece have some of the longest-living, healthiest people in the world, and beans are a big part of the equation. This recipe is simple Mediterranean brilliance!

1 pound dried beans, either gigantes beans (large Greek beans) or large lima beans
1½ cups chopped onion
1 cup diced celery, about 2 large stalks
1 cup olive oil
⅓ cup chopped garlic, about 15 cloves

¾ cup chopped fresh parsley
⅓ cup chopped fresh mint
1 tablespoon dried oregano, crushed between your hands
1 tablespoon salt
2 teaspoons freshly ground black pepper
2 cups crushed tomatoes
1 cup room-temperature water

Soak the dried beans for at least 7 hours. Drain and add the beans to a pot, covering with water by at least 2 inches. Boil for 50 minutes. Drain, reserving 2 cups of the cooking liquid.

Preheat the oven to 350°F.

Sauté the onions and celery in olive oil over medium-low heat until tender, about 15 minutes. Add the garlic and cook until it is soft, about 5 minutes. Stir in the herbs, salt, and pepper. Stir in the crushed tomatoes, and cook 5 more minutes. Add the reserved cooking liquid from the beans, and bring to a boil. Remove from the heat.

Layer the cooked beans evenly into a 13 × 9-inch baking dish, and pour the sauce over the top. Add 1 cup of room-temperature water, but don't stir. Bake, uncovered, for 2 hours, stirring every 30 minutes or so. Allow the beans to rest 15 to 30 minutes before serving.

> **Tip:** You can make the sauce well ahead of time so it's ready to go as soon as your beans have finished their initial cooking.

Frijoles de Olla
(excerpted from *Vegan Mexico*)

By Jason Wyrick

MAKES 6 CUPS OF BEANS

The quintessential pot of beans, frijoles de olla can be found simmering daily in most Mexican home kitchens. They are typically served directly from the cooking pot, usually an earthenware pot called an olla de barro, and they are served with the simmering stock. Beans are versatile, homey, tasty, and easy, and they get even better the next day. Frijoles de olla are often made with lard or bacon fat, so if you want a similar taste with your pot of beans, use the optional vegan shortening-liquid smoke-maple syrup mixture listed in the recipe.

1 pound dried beans (pinto, black, fava, garbanzo, or Peruvian)
1 small yellow or white onion, cut into ¼-inch dice
1½ to 2 teaspoons salt, divided
2 tablespoons plant-based shortening + 1 tablespoon maple syrup +
    1 teaspoon liquid smoke, combined, optional
3 to 4 tablespoons chili powder, optional
    (I prefer ancho powder with a dash of chipotle powder)
2 sprigs fresh epazote, chopped, or 1 tablespoon dried epazote, optional

Add the beans, 10 cups of water, onion, ½ teaspoon of the salt, and shortening combination, if using, to a 4-quart pot, and bring to a boil over high heat. Reduce the heat so that the water is simmering, and cook until the beans are just soft. This will take 1 to 2 hours, depending on the size and age of the beans. Add the remaining 1 to 1½ teaspoons salt and chili powder, if using, and cook until the stock is viscous, about 1 hour. If you are using the epazote, add it about 15 minutes before the beans are finished.

NOTE: Epazote is a long-leaf herb found in many traditional Mexican recipes. It is readily available at markets that specialize in Mexican cuisine.

Tofu "Chorizo"

By Mark Bittman, acclaimed food journalist,
fellow at the Union for Concerned Scientists, cookbook author

MAKES 4 SERVINGS

KF: Mark and I became friends when we realized we both love martinis and plant-based food, as well as having the shared belief in "progress, not perfection." As in, do what you can to make an impact on your health and the environment, but don't make yourself or anyone else crazy! I love how this recipe—like all of his recipes—is simple and without fuss. Because Mark is known as "the minimalist," he doesn't give super-detailed instructions, but rather loose guidelines and measurements. So adjust according to your taste!

Crumbled tofu, cooked until nearly all the water is driven out, produces a result that is very similar to ground meat and that takes on the flavor of whatever was cooked with it.

2 tablespoons olive oil	1 tablespoon chili powder
1 small onion, chopped	1 teaspoon ground cumin
3 garlic cloves, minced	⅛ teaspoon ground cinnamon
Salt to taste	1 teaspoon cider vinegar
Black pepper to taste	Chopped fresh cilantro for garnish
2 blocks firm tofu	Chopped green onions for garnish

Heat the oil in a large skillet over medium-high heat. Add the onion and garlic, and sprinkle with salt and pepper, stirring occasionally, until the vegetables soften, 3 to 5 minutes.

Crumble the tofu by hand into the pan. Cook, stirring and scraping the bottom of the skillet occasionally and adjusting heat as necessary, until the tofu browns and crisps as much or as little as you like, anywhere from 10 to 30 minutes.

Sprinkle with the chili powder, cumin, and cinnamon. Cook, stirring and continuing to scrape any browned bits from the bottom of the pan until the mixture is fragrant, 1 to 2 minutes. Stir in the vinegar and salt to taste. Remove from the heat and garnish with cilantro and green onions. Serve with warm corn tortillas or over rice.

Three Sisters' Sauté

By Lois Ellen Frank, PhD, New Mexico–based chef,
native food historian, from the Kiowa nation on her mother's side

MAKES 6 TO 8 SERVINGS

High in protein and nutrients and low in sugar and fat, corn, beans, and squash, also known as the Three Sisters, are considered by many tribal communities to be sacred gifts from the Great Spirit. The way these vegetables grow in the garden exemplifies this notion of interconnectedness, as do the complementary nutrients they provide. While this dish is good just as it is, my favorite way to eat the Three Sisters Sauté is with homemade corn tortillas.

Olive oil cooking spray
½ white onion, diced
2 garlic cloves, minced
2 cups organic, medium-size zucchini, cut into ¼-inch cubes
1½ cups cooked Anasazi, organic cranberry, organic pinto, or tepary beans or 1 (15-ounce) can organic pinto beans

1 cup corn kernels, preferably cut from roasted corn (see Note)
¼ cup chopped, roasted, and peeled New Mexico green chiles
½ teaspoon kosher or sea salt
⅛ teaspoon freshly ground black pepper

Spray the olive oil onto a cast-iron skillet to prevent sticking. Heat the skillet over medium heat until the oil is hot but not smoking. Sauté the onions for 2 minutes. Add the garlic and zucchini, and sauté for another 2 minutes. Add the cooked beans and corn and stir. Add the chopped green chiles, salt, and pepper, and cook for another 2 minutes, stirring constantly. Serve immediately with your favorite tortillas for a fantastic taco.

NOTE: For the roasted sweet corn, preheat oven to 350°F. Wet each ear of corn and place on a sheet tray. Add enough water to cover the bottom of the tray with ½ inch of water. Place in the oven and roast for approximately 10 minutes, remove from oven, turn over the ears of corn and roast for an additional 10 minutes. Remove from the oven, peel the husks and cut the kernels from the cob. Discard the husks and cob. Use as instructed in the recipe.

SNACKS AND SMALL BITES

Creamy Roasted Red Pepper and Cucumber Dip

 Kid Friendly

Recipe courtesy of Kite Hill

MAKES 1 CUP, 4 SERVINGS

KF: This creamy deliciousness made me forget any lingering attachment I had to dairy stuff. . . . Sigh.

8 ounces Kite Hill plain cream cheese
1 tablespoon za'atar
3 tablespoons peeled, diced cucumber
3 tablespoons diced roasted red pepper

Combine all the ingredients in a small bowl. Serve with pita chips, toasted bread, or on a bagel.

NOTE: Za'atar is a Middle Eastern spice mix made from dried thyme, sesame seeds, sumac, and salt.

Spinach Bacon Cream Cheese Dip Kid Friendly

By Jason Wyrick, executive chef of the Vegan Taste

MAKES 1 CUP, 4 SERVINGS

KF: Forget about serving humdrum hummus at a cocktail party; this dip will rock the taste buds!

2 strips Sweet Earth plant-based bacon, diced
1 tablespoon olive oil
1 small ancho chile, seeds and stem removed, optional
8 cups baby spinach leaves
6 roasted garlic cloves
¼ teaspoon salt, preferably mesquite-smoked salt
8 ounces Kite Hill chive cream cheese
½ teaspoon cracked black pepper

Over medium heat in a medium-size skillet, sauté the bacon in olive oil for 2 minutes, occasionally stirring. Remove from the pan, leaving as much oil in the pan as possible, and set aside. Return the pan to the heat, and add the ancho chile pieces, if using. Fry these for 30 seconds, remove from the pan, and set aside. Add the spinach to the pan and cook until completely wilted. Drain away any excess water in the pan. Smash the garlic cloves and salt into a paste.

In a mixing bowl, stir together the cream cheese, garlic paste, pepper, bacon pieces, and fried chile pieces, if using. Once the ingredients are thoroughly combined, stir in the spinach and serve.

Sikil Pak (excerpted from *Vegan Mexico*)

By Jason Wyrick

MAKES 1¾ CUPS, 6 SERVINGS

Sikil pak is a centuries-old Mayan pumpkin seed dip popular in Yucatán, but in modern restaurants, it's the rising star, replacing artisan guacamole as the haute cuisine Mexican dip. I don't care where it's served, in fancy restaurants or on the street, I will eat an entire bowl of sikil pak in a couple minutes if you let me. It's the heady creaminess of the pumpkin seeds combined with the slightly sweet, slightly tart roasted tomatillos that pulls me in. Serve with tortillas, tortilla chips, or sliced raw squash.

4 large tomatillos, husks removed
½ small white onion, cut into
   ¼-inch thick rings
3 garlic cloves, unpeeled

1 cup unsalted raw pepitas
1 teaspoon salt
¼ cup loosely packed fresh cilantro

Heat a skillet (preferably cast iron) over medium heat. Place the tomatillos, onion, and garlic in the skillet. As the tomatillos and onion rings blister and the garlic paper becomes dark brown, flip the ingredients and repeat. The garlic and onion will finish after 7 to 8 minutes and the tomatillos after 12 to 15 minutes. Place the tomatillos, onion, garlic, pepitas, salt, and cilantro in a blender and purée until completely smooth.

> ***Chef's tip:*** For a better texture, grind the ingredients in a molcajete (a Mexican mortar and pestle), starting with the onion, garlic, and salt until they become a rough paste. Next, add the pepitas and cilantro and continue smashing until the pepitas are creamy. Finish with the tomatillos, smashing them into the creamy pepitas until the sikil pak is mostly smooth. It's a lot more effort, but you will be well rewarded.

Buticha—Spicy Smashed Lemon Chickpeas
(excerpted from *Vegan Without Borders*)

Recipe by Robin Robertson

MAKES 4 SERVINGS

The Ethiopian dish called buticha is also known as "fasting eggs" because it resembles scrambled eggs in appearance. The flavor of this addictively delicious dish is like a lemony Ethiopian-spiced hummus (only better). Scoop it up with injera, the distinctive Ethiopian fermented flatbread, or with your favorite flatbread or crackers.

1½ cups (15-ounce can) cooked chickpeas, drained and rinsed

½ cup minced red onion

2 tablespoons chopped pickled jalapeños

1 garlic clove, minced

1 teaspoon grated fresh ginger

2 tablespoons (1 large lemon) freshly squeezed lemon juice

1 tablespoon olive oil

½ teaspoon prepared yellow mustard

½ teaspoon ground turmeric

¼ teaspoon ground cayenne

½ teaspoon salt

¼ teaspoon freshly ground black pepper

In a large, shallow bowl, mash the chickpeas well with a potato masher. Add the onion, jalapeños, garlic, and ginger, and combine. Alternatively, you can combine the ingredients in a food processor and pulse until chopped, but with a little texture remaining, then transfer to a bowl.

In a separate bowl, stir together the lemon juice, oil, mustard, turmeric, cayenne, salt, and pepper. Stir this mixture into the chickpea mixture, until evenly combined. If the mixture is too thick, you can stir a little water into it until you achieve your desired consistency. Cover and chill for at least 2 hours before serving to allow the flavors to meld. Serve chilled or at room temperature.

Roasted Brussels Sprouts with Hazelnut Chimichurri

By Daphne Cheng

MAKES 6 SERVINGS

KF: What a little punch of protein Brussels sprouts pack—30 percent protein! And Daphne makes them taste soooo delicious!

1½ pounds Brussels sprouts
½ cup plus 2 tablespoons olive oil, divided
2 teaspoons sea salt, divided
2 teaspoons black pepper, divided
1 cup packed chopped fresh parsley
½ cup toasted hazelnuts
½ cup packed chopped fresh cilantro
¼ cup red wine vinegar
1 garlic clove
Fresh basil or parsley as a garnish, optional

Preheat the oven to 425°F.

Slice the ends off the sprouts, then cut them in half. Toss the sprouts in 2 tablespoons of olive oil, 1 teaspoon of salt, and 1 teaspoon of black pepper. Spread onto a baking sheet and roast until the sprouts are browned, 15 to 20 minutes. Remove from the oven and season with salt and pepper to taste.

In a food processor or blender, puree the parsley, hazelnuts, cilantro, vinegar, garlic, ½ cup of olive oil, 1 teaspoon of salt, and 1 teaspoon of black pepper. Toss the sprouts in this mix and serve. Garnish with minced fresh basil or parsley, if you like.

Spiced Chickpeas
(excerpted from *Crossroads Cookbook*)

By Tal Ronnen, executive chef of Crossroads Kitchen,
plant-based powerhouse chef

MAKES 4 SERVINGS

KF: Tal is one of my best friends, so I have to brag on him for a minute: he's cooked for Oprah, Ellen and Portia, a slew of other celebrities and athletes who come into his super-sceney restaurant in Los Angeles, and he's been featured in a gazillion food magazines with rave reviews. He's a master at creating plant-based food that you don't even realize is plant based, and he's winning people over to animal-free food, one dish at a time!

With high levels of fiber and protein, there's no question that chickpeas are good for you. Sadly, though, they often fall short in the flavor department, ending up bland or, even worse, mealy. Scot and I are huge lovers of spicy food, so we tinkered around with ideas until we produced this dish, which packs a powerful punch of cumin, cayenne, and red pepper flakes. The marinara sauce added at the end gives the chickpeas a terra-cotta hue.

These spiced chickpeas pair well with flatbreads, rice, and even potato dishes. For a crunchy snack, season the chickpeas as directed and roast until dry on the outside and slightly tender in the middle, 30 to 35 minutes.

3 cups cooked, rinsed chickpeas
1 teaspoon ground cumin
1 teaspoon red pepper flakes
½ teaspoon cayenne pepper
½ teaspoon kosher salt
½ teaspoon freshly ground
　black pepper
6 tablespoons grapeseed oil, or
　oil of your choice, divided

½ shallot, minced
2 garlic cloves, minced
Juice of ½ lemon
1 tablespoon dry sherry
1 cup marinara sauce
Chopped flat-leaf parsley,
　for garnish

Preheat the oven to 425°F.

In a mixing bowl, combine the chickpeas, cumin, red pepper flakes, cayenne, salt, black pepper, and ¼ cup of the oil until thoroughly mixed together. Spread the chickpeas onto a baking sheet in a single layer. Roast, shaking the pan every 5 minutes or so, for 25 minutes, until the chickpeas are firm and dry. Set the chickpeas aside to cool.

Heat a large skillet over medium heat and add the remaining 2 tablespoons of oil. When the oil is hot, add the shallots and garlic, and cook for 2 minutes. Add the chickpeas and stir, until the chickpeas are hot. Stir in the lemon juice, sherry, and marinara sauce and cook until the sauce is hot, about 2 minutes.

Mound the chickpeas in a bowl, top with chopped parsley, and serve warm.

Tofu Marinated in Tealeaf Brine

By Ju Lan Bloom, KF's friend in China
who makes to-die-for local food

MAKES 4 SERVINGS

When I was a young student in Shanghai, my mom always made tofu in tealeaf brine during the winter. It was a snack for us that we brought to school.

3 tablespoons green tea leaves

5 whole star anise

5 whole cloves

3 (3- to 4-inch) cinnamon sticks

1 tablespoon whole black
   peppercorns

3 pieces dry orange peel

1 teaspoon salt

3 thin slices ginger

2 tablespoons sake

3 chives

5 tablespoons dark soy sauce

2 teaspoons granulated sugar

1 pound extra-firm tofu

Sesame oil, optional

Chopped cilantro, optional

Add all the ingredients, save for the tofu, to a pot with 6 cups of water, and bring to a boil. Reduce the heat to medium-low, and simmer for 20 minutes. Add the extra-firm tofu to the pot and cook for 10 to 15 minutes. Remove from the heat, transfer to the refrigerator once cool, and let the tofu marinate in the brine for 8 to 12 hours.

To serve, remove the tofu from the brine and cut into small pieces. Eat as is, or toss with sesame oil and chopped cilantro.

Chile Lime Peanuts

Recipe by Jason Wyrick

MAKES 1 CUP, 4 SERVINGS

Chile lime peanuts aren't just a classic Mexican bar food; they're also a protein-rich snack. These peanuts are little flavor bombs. A little bit goes a very long way. You can vary the heat on these by using different types of chili powders. Ancho chili powder will give a mild, caramel spiciness, chipotle powder will bring the heat and add a smokiness to the dish, while those of you who love the extremes of spicy food can make this with chile pequin powder, or even a dash of ghost chile powder.

1 cup unsalted raw peanuts, shelled
1 teaspoon olive oil
⅓ teaspoon sea salt
½ teaspoon chili powder (I prefer chipotle powder)
¼ teaspoon freshly ground black pepper
Juice of 1 lime

Cook the peanuts in a wide skillet over medium heat in the olive oil until lightly browned, about 5 minutes. Remove from the heat and immediately toss with the salt, chili powder, and pepper. Place in a bowl and sprinkle the lime juice on top.

Cultured Cashew Cheese

Recipe by Jason Wyrick

MAKES 1 CUP

KF: You can make your own cheese—joy!!!

This is a simple cultured cashew cheese, aged in a fashion similar to that of a dairy cheese. That culturing and aging creates a flavor profile surprisingly similar to a quick-aged dairy cheese, and it is well worth the wait. You can use this after a day as the base for creamy sauces or as a spread, or you can age it for weeks, or even months, to create a hard cheese that can be sliced or grated. This recipe is the base recipe, but you can add other flavor components such as minced chives, shaved truffles, peppercorns, minced rosemary, garlic, or whatever you are in the mood for at the time.

2 cups cashews, soaked for 6 to 8 hours, then drained and rinsed

¼ teaspoon sea salt

2 probiotic capsules or ¼ cup nondairy unsweetened yogurt

Add the cashews and salt to a blender and open up the probiotic capsules and pour the powder into the blender. Alternatively, you can use nondairy yogurt instead of the capsules to create the cheese culture. Blend the mix together until smooth. Add any other flavoring ingredients at this point, if using. Scoop into cheesecloth and tie it closed. Ideally, you want to suspend the cheesecloth bag from something, like a coat hanger, to give the cashew cheese time to dry. If you can't hang it, place it on a wire rack or simply on a plate as a last resort. Let this sit for 12 hours, then transfer it to the refrigerator, and age at least 12 more hours. This will produce a spreadable cashew cream cheese that you can also use as the base for cream sauces. If you let this age three days, the cheese flavor will intensify, and the cheese will thicken. If you age it for a week, you can create a soft sliceable cream cheese. Don't stop there, though. Age it for three to four months, and you'll have a hard cheese reminiscent of Parmesan that can be grated.

Make it into pasta Alfredo: Puree ½ cup of the Cultured Cashew Cheese, aged only one day, with 2 garlic cloves, ¼ cup unsweetened almond milk, and salt to taste. Toss with your favorite cooked pasta, and garnish with chopped chives and freshly ground black pepper.

Make it into a mezze platter: Age the cheese one week, then mold it into a palm-size cheese wheel and garnish with minced fresh rosemary. Serve on a platter with olives of your choice, roasted red pepper strips, hummus, and sliced bread for a light lunch or an appetizer.

DESSERTS

Avocado Chocolate Mousse Crunch

Recipe by Jason Wyrick, executive chef of the Vegan Taste

MAKES 2 SERVINGS

I was skeptical of avocado chocolate mousse when I first heard about it years ago, but I'm willing to try just about anything plant based. That first bite changed my mind, and I have been a fan ever since. You really can't taste the avocado, but the texture it lends is like a firm cream, exactly what you want from a mousse. Add some dried cherries, dates, and nuts, and you've got a dessert that manages to be healthy and taste decadent at the same time. Even better, it only takes a couple of minutes of work. The hard part is staring at the refrigerator waiting for the mousse to set!

The Mousse

2 ripe avocados, peeled and pitted
½ cup cocoa powder
¼ cup agave syrup
1 teaspoon almond extract
⅛ teaspoon salt

The Crunch

4 dried cherries, chopped
1 pitted date, chopped
2 tablespoons toasted slivered
   almonds
1 tablespoon chopped roasted
   salted peanuts

In a food processor, whip together all the ingredients for the mousse until smooth. Chill the mousse for at least 3 hours, and up to 24 hours, before serving. Transfer to two serving cups and sprinkle all the Crunch ingredients on top.

Pink Peppercorn Peanut Brittle

Recipe by Jason Wyrick

MAKES 4 SERVINGS

Even though peanut brittle is high in protein, that's not what I'm thinking when I'm eating it. What I'm really thinking is, "Please sir, can I have another?" This is my slightly gourmet version of it, using smoked salt and pink peppercorns, and, unlike a lot of other peanut brittles, this does not utilize corn syrup. If you just want a straight-up peanut brittle without the fancy components, you can replace the smoked salt with regular salt and skip the pink peppercorns.

1 cup granulated sugar, preferably
   turbinado or demerara sugar
¼ teaspoon smoked salt
1½ cups roasted salted peanuts
   (for a flavor explosion, use
   Chile Lime Peanuts, page 215)
1 tablespoon nondairy butter
½ teaspoon vanilla extract
Pinch cinnamon
1 teaspoon lightly crushed pink
   peppercorns
⅛ teaspoon baking soda

Lightly oil, with oil of your choice, a baking sheet or silicon mat, and set it aside.

In a medium-size heavy saucepan or iron skillet over medium heat, combine the sugar, salt, and ¾ cup of water, stirring until the sugar dissolves. Adjust the heat until it comes to a slow simmer, and keep the mix at a slow simmer the whole time it is on the stove. Gently stir occasionally until the mix turns an amber color. This will take 10 to 15 minutes.

As soon as it turns an amber color, immediately remove from the heat, and quickly stir in the peanuts, nondairy butter, vanilla extract, cinnamon, peppercorns, and baking soda. Continue stirring until the mixture turns glossy. Transfer this to the baking sheet or mat and spread it out. Let the mix sit for at least 20 minutes, until it has hardened and turned brittle.

NOTE: To make this kid-friendly, omit the pink peppercorns.

Black Bean Brownies with Toasted Pepitas Kid Friendly

Recipe by Jason Wyrick

MAKES 9 SERVINGS

Beans in dessert? Inconceivable! Or so I thought until I tried my first black bean brownies. The black beans and chocolate are natural pairs. Add chipotle chiles for a sweet and spicy dessert, and I'm in love.

⅓ cup whole wheat pastry flour, or coarsely ground rolled oats for a gluten-free option

¼ cup cocoa powder

¾ teaspoon baking powder

¼ teaspoon salt

¼ to ½ teaspoon chipotle powder, optional

½ cup maple syrup

¼ cup coconut oil, plus more for greasing the pan

1½ cups (14-ounce can) cooked black beans, drained and rinsed

2 teaspoons vanilla or almond extract

¾ cup nondairy chocolate chips, divided

3 to 4 tablespoons toasted salted pepitas or peanuts

Heat the oven to 350°F.

In a mixing bowl, whisk together the flour, cocoa powder, baking powder, salt, and chipotle powder, if using. Transfer to a food processor, along with the maple syrup, coconut oil, black beans, and extract, and process until mostly smooth. Transfer back to the mixing bowl and stir in ½ cup of the chocolate chips.

Grease a 9 × 9-inch pan with coconut oil, and spread the brownie batter inside. Spread the remaining chocolate chips and pepitas or peanuts on top, and pat them down lightly into the brownies. Bake the brownies for 17 minutes, then let them cool for at least 10 minutes before serving.

Chia Chai Blueberry Pudding Parfaits

Recipe by Jason Wyrick

MAKES 4 SERVINGS

I love simple desserts that are sweet but not overly so. This easy chia seed parfait is loaded with good protein from the seeds, redolent of all the best flavors of chai, and eminently refreshing with the addition of fresh blueberries. It's a feel-good dessert for both your body and your palate.

1 cup almond milk, or coconut milk for a richer dessert

2 containers (5.3 ounces each) nondairy vanilla yogurt

1 tablespoon agave syrup, optional

¼ teaspoon ground cardamom

¼ teaspoon ground cinnamon

Pinch of ground cloves

Pinch of black pepper

Pinch of salt

¼ cup chia seeds

½ cup fresh blueberries

¼ cup toasted slivered almonds

In a mixing bowl, whip together the nondairy milk, yogurt, syrup (if using), cardamom, cinnamon, cloves, pepper, and salt. Stir in the chia seeds. Cover and refrigerate for 6 to 8 hours.

Spoon into small glasses, top with fresh blueberries, and finish with toasted almonds.

CHAPTER 14

Become an Activist
in the Revolution

Plant protein is growing faster than animal protein.
For us, we want to be where the consumer is.
— Tom Hayes, CEO of Tyson Foods

If you were on the fence about a plant-based diet, we hope the information and recipes in this book have emboldened you to make the switch. Opting out of animal protein is the best way to help the environment, the economy, and your health.

But don't stop there!

As Gandhi said, "You must be the change you want to see in the world." Replacing animal protein in your diet will improve your health, but it won't improve your neighbor's heart disease or your aunt's diabetes. Plants will reduce your carbon footprint, but they won't affect Mom and Dad's. If you're feeling connected to this movement, spread the word, so that we can begin to end our dependence on dirty protein, one kitchen at a time.

When you're done reading this book, please give it to your friends, family members, and coworkers. Become an expert by reading other excellent books on plant-based nutrition, as well as online resources such as the Good Food Institute blog at gfi.org, Dr. Michael Greger's invaluable website, www.nutritionfacts.org, and Dr. Neal Barnard's blog over at the Physicians Committee for Responsible Medicine (www.pcrm.org). In the meantime, here are some tips for convincing others to join the movement.

BE KNOWLEDGEABLE TO FIGHT THE MYTHS

Albert Einstein is reported to have quipped, "If the facts don't fit the theory, change the facts." As long as the animal food industry is around, it will continue to distort and manipulate facts to generate uncertainty. We saw the exact same tactics employed by the tobacco industry to combat health and regulatory legislation. Key to the industry's tactics are age-old myths about plant-based eating that never seem to die. It's up to you to refute them. When Uncle Joe cracks jokes about your squash and white bean casserole at Thanksgiving dinner, smile (genuinely) and let him know in a very kind manner why you're eating this way. Don't let a bully get the best of you. You've researched this, and you're doing it for a whole bunch of really good reasons. Just let him know the one that's closest to your heart, and then move on.

We know there's a lot to remember, but you don't have to be a scholar on the subject. You just need to know enough to effectively discuss the merits of a clean protein diet so that you can pique people's curiosity and, more importantly, quell their concerns. Here's a quick guide to help you counter the most common myths skeptics raise.

Myth 1: Plant-based eaters don't get enough protein. This one is easy! By now you know that just about *all whole plant–based foods have protein.* If you really want to make a point to Uncle Joe, say something like, "I didn't realize that protein deficiency was an issue in the United States. Is there a protein deficiency epidemic I wasn't aware of?" Be sure to wait for an answer—silence is your friend, and you want Joe to realize for himself that he doesn't know anyone who is suffering from a protein deficiency.

As a basic principle, you want to engage in a conversation, not a monologue. We're just giving you some ideas of things to say, but do, of course, leave room for listening as well.

Once you have Joe thinking about the lack of a protein deficiency epidemic in the United States, you might want to point out that heart disease, obesity, diabetes—those are the health issues that are plaguing Americans, not protein deficiency.

You might also say something like, "Well, Uncle Joe, according to a 2013 study in the *Journal of the Academy of Nutrition and Dietetics,* plant-based eaters on average receive 70 percent more protein than the minimum recommended intake." You can also tell him that, nationwide, there's no one who is protein deficient who is eating enough food.

You might also tell Joe that broccoli has more protein per calorie than steak, that spinach has just as much protein per calorie as fish and chicken. Then you can remind him about top mixed-martial-arts fighters Mac Danzig, Jake Shields, and James Wilks—all vegans. Tell him about Scott Jurek, who broke the world record for the fastest Appalachian Trail run. Tell him about the football player David Carter, who attributes his strength and stamina to a plant-based diet. All of these athletes pushed their bodies to the max and have no problem obtaining all the protein they needed from plants.

At this point your uncle might be getting uncomfortable. The goal here is not to shame someone or to "win" an argument; you only want to disabuse him of old and outdated notions. You can politely move on after mentioning how plant-based eaters take in all the complete proteins they need but that meat-eaters consume *dangerous* protein. Tell him that animal protein is associated with higher rates of heart disease, kidney disease, inflammatory bowel disease, inflammatory arthritis, colon cancer, and many other chronic diseases. Say it with a smile, because, after all, this is exciting and empowering stuff. And then offer him a bite of your Gardein or Beyond Meat, Hungry Planet, or Tofurky, and he'll realize how delicious the clean protein alternatives can be.

Myth 2: There is no evidence that a plant-based diet is healthy. This one is easy to respond to by just having a few facts tucked up your sleeve. Just let it be known that an overwhelming number of clinical trials have proven that a plant-based diet can prevent, arrest, or even reverse chronic disease, especially heart disease and diabetes. Tell him that the Academy of Nutrition and Dietetics reviewed all of the science that exists on vegetarian and vegan diets and determined that people who eat no meat at all are the healthiest populations in the country. The academy also declared that plant-based diets are healthy for all people at all ages, including for nursing mothers and infants.

You might also discuss the work of Drs. Dean Ornish and Caldwell Esselstyn, who have taken patients with end-stage heart disease and completely reversed their prognosis. Not managed, not controlled, but *cured*. Studies involving hundreds of thousands of people have repeatedly proven that eating fewer animal products is directly correlated with a longer life and lower risk of chronic disease. If the myth-insister mentions a study that shows meat, fish, eggs, or dairy are healthy, tell him to follow the money. Chances are that study was funded by the animal food industry or its methodology is questionable. (There are numerous studies cited in this book, so choose your favorites and keep them at the ready when someone needs proof of what you're saying.) Lastly, recommend they watch *Forks over Knives* on Netflix; it's chock full of great health information and it's easy to understand and, er, digest.

Myth 3: People who don't eat animal protein are frail. This myth is especially insidious. First, explain to the person challenging you that plant eaters might appear thin because they are the *only* demographic in America at an ideal body weight. After sifting through data from more than 60,000 men and women, Loma Linda University researchers found that the average body mass index for people who consume no animal products was 23.6 (between 18.5 and 24.9 is considered ideal, between 25 and 29.9 overweight, and over 30 obese). Meat-eaters averaged a 28.8—close to obese. You can say with confidence, "No, I'm not frail—I'm actually really healthy." (And then invite him to go hiking or running with you!)

Your aunt may chime in that a plant-based diet may be healthy for adults, but children need a more robust diet to fuel their growth. Sorry, Aunt Patty, but the opposite is true. Studies show that children raised on a clean protein diet are not just leaner than children who grow up on the standard American diet, they're *taller* too, by about an inch.

Myth 4: Clean protein is expensive. Many people believe that meat- and dairy-free products are a luxury that only rich people can afford. Even though taxpayers are heavily subsidizing the animal food industry, eating plant based on a budget is easy and affordable. Plant-based staples such as potatoes, brown rice, and beans are very cheap and keep for a long time. While fresh produce is best, frozen fruits and vegetables are cheap, nutritious, and keep indefinitely.

While pricier meat alternatives like Tofurky or Quorn are delicious, they are not necessary. You can easily substitute them for protein-rich beans, lentils, and tofu. Check out resources like www.forksoverknives.com for easy and inexpensive meal plans.

Myth 5: Not eating animal food is "extreme." When all else fails, skeptics will fall back on this doozy. Your uncle may mumble something about "eating everything in moderation" or that cutting out animal products is "too extreme." In response, just paraphrase this quote from Dr. Esselstyn: "Some people think the plant-based, whole-foods diet is extreme. Half a million people a year will have their chests opened up and a vein taken from their leg and sewn onto their coronary artery. Some people would call that extreme."

ASK FOR CLEAN, PLANT-BASED PROTEIN AT RESTAURANTS

Imagine this (likely) scenario: A few weeks after you've switched to a mostly plant-based diet, you visit your favorite restaurant with your friends. You glance at the menu, and the entrees are beef, chicken, pork, and fish. Now what? If you ask your waiter for plant-based options, he might suggest ordering a side of grilled vegetables and a baked potato. Those are certainly fine options, but restaurants can do better, and they should if they want to keep up with the changing market. You might drop this doozy to the manager or chef: when given a choice, an astounding 37 percent of the country is choosing to eat veg when dining out. This is no longer a phenomenon you'll see only in one of the coastal cities; this is happening in towns and cities everywhere, especially among young people (a.k.a. the future consumers that restaurants surely want to hold on to). The better the menu offerings, the more diners will seek them out. Most people grew up accustomed to seeing protein at the center of their plates, and they've come to expect it. If you're spending your hard-earned money at a restaurant, you deserve a hearty meal. You deserve to feel happy. You deserve to feel full. And psychologically speaking, that means you'll enjoy the meal more if it's clean protein centric. Restaurateurs need to know that, so feel free to tell them.

Ask your waiter, "What do you have that is plant-based protein?" Be courteous, but phrase the question with the expectation that the restaurant *should* offer it. If you have friends who frequent that restaurant, have them ask the same question. Restaurateurs are generally embarrassed when they fail to accommodate their customers. Managers are always asking their service staff about customer requests so they can better serve them; so don't be surprised if a plant-based option appears quickly.

Remember to always be polite and respectful, even if they have nothing but steak, chicken, pork, and fish. If they do not offer clean, plant-based protein, you can say, "Hey, I truly love coming to your restaurant. I love the atmosphere and everyone who works here, but I'm disappointed that you don't have more plant-based options. I would love to spend my money here, but I'm afraid I'm going to go elsewhere so that I can eat something hearty like everyone else." Ask to speak to the manager or chef—oftentimes they can whip something up for you, even if it's not on the menu. Afterward, thank the staff profusely. Tip well. Love them up on social media. The more you show your gratitude, the more likely restaurants are to make plant-based entrées permanent.

Be sure to ask for plant protein even when you know the answer is no. Likewise, when you're flying, ask the flight attendants if they have soy or almond milk for your coffee, even if you know they don't. The point is to keep reminding corporations that they are not accommodating all of their customers. They listen. For example, Starbucks has a web page where customers can make requests, and in 2016 the corporation announced that it was introducing almond milk after overwhelming customer demand.

Finally, don't be afraid to ask in the unlikeliest of places! One of Kathy's favorite restaurants is Lucky's Steakhouse in Santa

Barbara. They have a fantastic atmosphere and the most divine martinis, and Kathy loves coming with her friends. But all she could eat was a baked potato and a side of broccoli. One day she took the manager aside.

"Leonard," she said. "I absolutely love coming here, but you don't have any plant-based entrees. Can't you add one to the menu?"

"Well, this isn't a vegetarian restaurant," Leonard replied. "This is a steak house."

"I understand that, I really do. I have no problem with my friends ordering steaks. But I want to give you my money. Look at the margins. Tofu and seitan are so inexpensive, and so are plant-protein burgers . . . and they all keep for a long time, and it's as easy (or easier) to make than chicken or steak. I'd be so incredibly grateful if you'd just try it!"

Kathy kept at it, and eventually Lucky's tested a plant-based protein entrée. It is a business, after all, and it wants to please its customers. For the first time, Lucky's Steakhouse introduced a tofu option with the same famous sauce used on its sea bass. Believe it or not, tofu is now one of its most popular dishes! It just recently added a Hungry Planet burger, and diners seem to love that it's high in protein and low in calories and fat. Always remember that restaurants want to please their customers. They are not ideologically driven. As clean, plant-based diets become increasingly popular, restaurant owners will increasingly know they can't get away with sides of French fries and Brussels sprouts.

Craig's Restaurant in Los Angeles perfectly embodies how restaurants are adapting to customer demand. Its menu has your typical American options, including chicken parmigiana, whitefish piccata, lamb chops, and the 18-ounce prime rib-eye steak. But featured prominently on the menu is the vegan section. You can order delicious dishes like vegan chicken parmigiana, or spaghetti squash primavera, or vegan spaghetti Bolognese. Just recently it added an astoundingly delicious ice-cream made from cashew milk, and its customers responded so positively—begging to take home pints of it at the end of their meals—that now it's gone into the ice-cream business, as well! The restaurant's founder, Craig Susser, told the *New York Times* that he simply wants to accommodate plant-based customers: "I'm willing to do anything. I want them here, and I want them happy."

POST YOUR RECIPES ON SOCIAL MEDIA

Many people switch to plant-based diets to improve their health or to take a stand against animal cruelty. Both are excellent goals, but here's another great reason: the food tastes amazing!

Try posting your favorite recipes on Facebook, Twitter, Instagram, and other social media platforms. (If you are posting someone else's recipe, be sure to tag him or her and get permission where necessary.) Most important, begin with high-quality photos. We don't mean you need to be a professional photographer. But take pictures of the food that would look sumptuous to you, if you were the one perusing. No one is going to want to try a new dish if the food looks grey, fuzzy, or slimy with too much oil caught in a flash. Cell phones are just fine, especially if you use an app that allows you to edit efficiently. Or if you're really serious about becoming a clean protein activist, you could certainly invest in a quality camera that can most effectively capture your brilliant red tomatoes and splendid yellow squash. Experiment with different angles and backgrounds to make your recipes stand out in cluttered news feeds.

Emphasize how quick and easy your meals are. Ideally, only post meals that take thirty minutes or less to prepare. The last thing your followers want to see is a complicated meal that requires a mountain of obscure ingredients and an entire evening to cook. You want to demonstrate to your friends and family that plant-based meals are *easy* and *fast*. Stick to common ingredients and spices that are available at any grocery store. (Unless of course, exquisitely made haute cuisine is your thing; if that's the case, celebrate and share your culinary genius!)

Try featuring recipes that look and taste like your friends' favorite non-plant-based dishes. Show them photos of your decadent mac and cheese dish that uses cashews instead of Cheddar, or that delicious pesto sauce whipped together with basil, almonds, and fresh garlic. Avoid posting too many recipes that look "stereotypically" plant based, such as plain rice and beans or blocks of unseasoned tofu. (Blah. Yuck.) People raised on the standard American diet want to see that plant-based meals look just like—or better than—their old mainstays while being just as delicious.

Of course, the best way to share recipes is to cook them for your friends! The most effective way to bring your friends into the movement is to demonstrate how mouthwateringly good clean protein meals can be. Everyone wants to be healthier and help animals, but everyone wants to enjoy their food, too. Feeding your friends bland, tasteless meals will only reinforce bad stereotypes and turn them away.

BE ENTREPRENEURIAL—INVEST IN OR START YOUR OWN BUSINESS

There has never been a better time for plant-based products and restaurants!

Just ask twenty-nine-year-old Chloe Coscarelli, founder of the vegan fast-casual restaurant By Chloe, located in downtown New York. After winning the Food Network's *Cupcake Wars,* Chloe realized that plant-based foods weren't just scrumptious— many people outright preferred animal-free fare to traditional animal-based food. Her friends thought she was crazy to pack her menu with plant-based selections such as the quinoa taco salad, mac and cheese with a sweet potato cashew sauce, and guac burgers. But when Chloe's cheerful and hip restaurant opened its doors, the line was more than a block long, and it continues to pack the house day in and day out.

Meanwhile, the restaurateur Ravi DeRossi decided in 2016 to turn his ubersuccessful cocktail bar empire entirely plant based. Despite running fifteen highly profitable New York hot spots including the Bourgeois Pig, famous for its cheese plates, DeRossi decided that change was necessary. "If we're going to do something to help this planet, it needs to start," he told the website Eater. "It needs to be me not just preaching, but me just doing it. You don't realize that the average restaurateur does three times more destruction [to the environment] than the average person."

Coscarelli and DeRossi have proved that restaurants not serving animal foods are not just for vegans. When the food is good, everyone will eat it. Launched in 2013, Crossroads Kitchen in LA was one of the first restaurants to feature gorgeous Mediterranean fare, sans the fish and feta. Tal Ronnen, the founder and executive chef, was written up and celebrated as one of the most creative chefs in the country, and Crossroads was voted the best new hot spot to enjoy great food and celebrity sightings. Yet only a very small fraction of its customers consider themselves solely plant-based eaters; the vast majority simply want good food.

In addition to helping the environment and reducing cruelty in the food system, plant-based restaurants are also moneymakers. Once only seen on the trendiest city blocks, plant-based restaurants have exploded into a multibillion-dollar industry. Thanks to delicious food and low costs compared to traditional food providers—some restaurants report as much as 30 percent reduced food costs—plant-based restaurants are appearing in the unlikeliest of places. In July 2016, North Dakota's first vegan restaurant, Green House Café, opened in Fargo. Brooklyn and Los Angeles are one thing, but a restaurant in North Dakota that doesn't serve meat is like a ski shop in Barbados. Ranching is one of the most important industries in the state, and beef cattle outnumber humans by nearly three to one. And yet the restaurant is thriving. As beef consumption continues to decline nationwide, restaurants like Green House Café will continue to multiply.

Nicknamed "Cowtown," Fort Worth, Texas, is the heart of cattle country. The home of slaughterhouses and 72-ounce steaks, Fort Worth is perhaps the least likely place for a plant-based restaurant to succeed. Yet Spiral Diner, Fort Worth's first vegan restaurant, is wildly popular. In fact, it recently opened its third location. Visitors to Spiral Diner often wind their way from the stockyards, the epicenter of the Midwest cattle trade during the nineteenth century. In a city famous for its beef, Spiral Diner attracts residents from all walks of life to delicious plant-based cuisine, from businesspeople to seniors to tattooed hipsters in skinny jeans. (A nod here to Dan Buettner for helping to "Blue Zone" Fort Worth by working with the city to make healthy eating easier in the city.)

If they can make it work in Fargo and Fort Worth, you can do it in your hometown. And it doesn't have to be 100 percent plant based; any step away from animal foods and toward cleaner protein is a positive move. For interested entrepreneurs, check out www. happycow.net for a thorough database of plant-based restaurants or places that at least serve a few dishes so that everyone—vegan or committed carnivore—can eat well. We think that once people try some good plant-based food, they will see there is nothing to miss, and they'll lean even further. So, how well represented is your town? As the clean protein movement continues to win people over from coast to coast, now is the time to get in on the ground floor!

GET POLITICAL

Given all we know about how the government sets food policy, effective change is much more likely to start in kitchens and dining rooms than in the halls of Congress. As we saw in Chapter 4, the USDA publishes the influential *Dietary Guidelines,* which affects what kids eat in schools, among other far-reaching government programs. Unsurprisingly, the process is entirely hamstrung by animal agriculture lobbyists, who ensure the guidelines do not advocate plant-based eating.

There are ways to fight fire with fire. You can donate money to an organization which works to educate people on why a plant based diet is healthy, like NutritionFacts.org. Or if you're more interested in the business side of things, the Good Food Institute employs a team of scientists, entrepreneurs, lawyers, and lobbyists, all of whom are laser focused on using markets and food technology to transform our food system away from factory-farmed animal products and toward clean meat and plant-based alternatives.

You might also think about the Physicians Committee for Responsible Medicine, which was founded by Dr. Neal Barnard in 1985 and boasts more than 150,000 members. PCRM is devoted to changing the way health-care professionals approach heart disease, diabetes, obesity, and cancer. PCRM advocates that medical schools introduce more nutrition classes so that chronic disease may finally be seen as a consequence of poor diet. PCRM also works with Congress to push farm subsidy reform, nutritional reform for school lunches and food stamp programs, and many other crucial campaigns. To fight the onslaught of animal food industry money in government, donating to organizations like PCRM is an excellent first step.

Next, educate yourself. How have your elected representatives voted on issues concerning nutrition, health care, and the environment? For now it is difficult to see how lawmakers stand on plant-based nutrition issues, mainly because these bills never make it through Congress. Animal industry lobbyists have guaranteed that bills providing funding for plant-based clinical trials or education for doctors will never see the light of day. However, the Humane Society Legislative Fund has a scorecard where you can see how your representatives voted on animal agriculture issues. Based on that score, you can get a basic idea about their stance on reducing our dependence on animal products.

You don't need to hire a high-powered lobbyist to have your voice heard. Write a letter, call, or ask for a meeting with your representative or senator. (They actually take meetings, or at least someone in their office will. Your thoughts and concerns are always taken into account!) Tell them that our top causes of death are preventable with sensible dietary changes, and we need our government to make this known to the public by preventing animal industry lobbyists from influencing the *Dietary Guidelines*. Then call and write to your state legislators (who they are is easy to Google by simply entering in "senator/representative" and your state, and their contact information will also be provided online), who may be in a better position to pass effective laws on a local level. Use social media and get your friends and family to do the same. If there is going to be change, our representatives need to know that the public is clamoring for it.

Write letters to your local papers—a well-written and concise letter to the editor can influence thousands of people. Even if your words aren't printed, enough likeminded letters from your friends can convince newspaper editors that their audience is interested in clean protein issues. Stay engaged on social media; use the hashtag #cleanprotein or #cleanproteinrevolution. As many as 60 percent of Americans receive their news from social media, so what shows up on news feeds is more important than ever. Don't spam, but be sure to post action alerts from reputable organizations on a regular basis. The more people are aware of the issues, the more likely we can do something about them.

Finally, remember that nothing is more important than face-to-face conversations. Host delicious plant-based dinner parties and explain to your friends why this stuff is so important (and exciting)!

TALK TO YOUR DOCTOR

Maybe it's the white coat, but, when doctors talk, too many of us are afraid to question what they say. After all, it's not fun watching your doctor's eyes roll when you ask how you can reverse heart disease and diabetes by moving away from meat, dairy, and eggs. Too many people give up and say, "Well, I thought about cutting out all animal products, but my doctor said it wouldn't help."

Don't be afraid. Doctors are not infallible. Only a quarter of medical schools offer even a single dedicated nutrition course. One doctor friend of ours remembers that when he applied to medical school, an administrator told him that "nutrition is superfluous to human health." While he was a student, he was offered steak dinners and other perks from pharmaceutical companies. From day one, doctors are conditioned to believe that our leading causes of death are inevitable and can only be managed with drugs and surgery. While modern medicine can miraculously cure and prevent many conditions once thought to be a death sentence—and many doctors and surgeons are bona fide miracle workers—nutrition remains a blind spot.

Don't be afraid to ask your doctor questions. The airwaves are full of television ads imploring you to "ask your doctor" about this or that medication. Why not take a page out of Pfizer's playbook and ask your doctor whether a plant-based diet is right for you? If she is skeptical, ask her to read the latest nutritional studies, or give her a copy of this book. (Again, you will find lots of references herein.) Prove to her that you can lower your cholesterol and blood pressure naturally simply by cutting out animal protein. While you should always make major changes to your lifestyle in consultation with medical professionals, sometimes doctors need to see the incredible power of clean protein right up close. If it works for you, why can't it work for their other patients?

Learn to ask the right questions. If you have high cholesterol or blood pressure, it is possible that medication is necessary to lower your risk of heart attack or stroke, but be sure to ask your doctor about dietary options. Ask her how much of a cholesterol drop you can expect from replacing meat, eggs, and dairy with beans, grains, and veggies. Ask her what sorts of foods you should be eating for cancer prevention. Ask her about protein. If your doctor scoffs or assures you that dietary changes are useless, then consider switching to another provider. You want someone who understands the power of diet as well as the benefits and drawbacks of modern medicine.

If you are looking for a new doctor, ask your insurance provider for a recommendation in their database of someone who incorporates plant-based nutrition in their practice. While you should always see a fully licensed health-care professional, choosing a doctor, dietician, or physician's assistant with an understanding of plant-based eating can mean the difference between good health and chronic disease. If your current doctor has helped you discover the power of plants, be sure to love her up on social media and spread the word!

LOOK AND ACT THE CHANGE

Begin by taking good care of yourself, attending to your health, and presenting your best self as an example of what this shift looks like. Just because a diet is plant based does not mean it is healthy—there are lots of cookies and chips that have no animal stuff in them, after all; but eating junk food is not going to show off what clean protein looks like. Embody the shift in whatever way you think elevates the message. Eat healthfully, dress your best, and exercise to stay fit. People will eat like you to look like you!

Be respectful of others. One terrible stereotype of activists is that people who don't eat meat are elitist know-it-alls. Don't play into that stereotype. If you are at a restaurant with friends, don't complain when they order steak or chicken. Don't tut-tut moms and dads who give their children milk. It's great to be provocative, but don't be a pain. If you're in an argument with a relative at Thanksgiving, don't get angry if he's hell-bent on singing the praises of the leg he's eating. Don't get angry if he takes a demonstrably large bite just to show you his scorn when you riff about why you like clean protein. You may not be able to change that relative, but everyone else at the table might well be persuaded by your calm, informed sharing and your lack of judgement.

If someone asks you a silly or deliberately hostile question, never respond with sarcasm. For example, say a friend blurts, "But everyone knows that we need lots of protein, but plants don't have any." Don't start with "Actually . . . " or "You're wrong." Instead, say, "That's a very common point you raise, but it turns out that plants contain plenty of protein." Be friendly and conversational. Be humble and offer information, not self-righteous lectures. No one has all the answers.

Finally, carry yourself with dignity and grace. You're going to confront trolls, whether on Twitter, Facebook, or at the Thanksgiving table after a few bottles of wine. You're not going to convince everyone. Remember that *any* step toward reducing animal product consumption is positive. Plenty of people will agree to give up meat but not cheese, milk but not eggs, pork but not chicken.

Small steps should be applauded, not chided. A small minority of activists believe you have to "go all in." No, you don't. While cutting out all animal products is ideal, it can take a while to get there. Most people have been eating the same way for decades. Every little step counts.

Epilogue: Two (Very Different) Views from the Future

It could go this way:

A hundred years from now the world is unrecognizable. We did not heed the rising tide of health crises and climate change and zoonotic diseases. Society as we know it is fraying at the seams. Our country is a sicker, darker, hungrier place.

We've known for years what caused this. The warning signs were all there, yet we did nothing. We saw our friends and family growing sicker, our air warmer, our seas higher. Antibiotics, which had been recklessly pumped into farm animals for more than a century, stopped working for humans, and people began dying from what used to be easily treatable infections. We knew the primary cause was a wasteful, polluting, and dangerous source of food, but we continued to pile it onto our plates.

Historians are surprised that twenty-first-century humans ignored the medical science linking meat consumption to degenerative diseases like cancer, heart disease, obesity, and diabetes. Anthropologists are less surprised, noting that mass industrialization made these foods cheap and ubiquitous and that millions of years of evolution had programmed the human body to crave

high-fat foods. Economists point to the enormous taxpayer subsidies that made selling unhealthy, unsustainable food extremely
profitable. Others point to the industry's giant PR machine with
tentacles extending into every corridor of power in Washington.
For too long, society was plagued by health problems and propped
up with drugs and expensive surgeries. Our economy was dependent on the profits generated by poor health. And in the fog of
ever-more potent pharmaceuticals, we remained blissfully unaware
of our doomed trajectory.

In the face of environmental studies revealing the gross inefficiency and polluting nature of animal protein, the world's governments did nothing. Rainforests were cut down to graze and feed
animals, releasing vast quantities of carbon dioxide that had been
safely stored by trees. More than half of the world's fresh water
was devoted to farm animal production. We watched the biodiversity of fish and coral disappear because of commercial fishing and
trawling operations. Torrential weather devastated cities and economies. Millions of people had their homes and lives destroyed. The
once-wealthy economies of North America and Europe collapsed
from the devastation of catastrophic weather that leveled city after
city with utter devastation.

Although many of our brightest minds denounced the com-
modification of animals, there was no universal cry of indignation.
The protestations remained weak and "elitist." There were no de-
nunciations from religious bodies, no mass boycotts of the largest
commodifiers—in short, no proportional response worthy of the
injustices that were being inflicted on animals, our health, our environment, and our economy. Just like the Mesopotamians, the
Mayans, and the Romans before us, our large and interconnected
world was susceptible to breakdown. We saw the signs. We were
warned. But we were hypnotized by the sway of Big Food. We
collaborated in our own demise.

A scary possibility, right? This future is entirely possible if we do not change course. Yet it is far from inevitable. The seas are rising, but they can stabilize. Our health is deteriorating, but chronic illness can be reversed. Our forests can be regrown. But we have to start now, because premonitions of this dark future can already be seen from the pig factories of China to the laboratories of the Centers for Disease Control and Prevention in Atlanta to the beetle-infested forests of Northern California to the ravaged Great Barrier Reef in Australia. The trajectory is already underway. This is not exaggerated or unreasonable—it is scientific reality.

But what if we turn the ship around, starting today? The result is a very different future. . . .

By midcentury, humans fully grasp the link between conventional animal protein and medical, economic, and environmental catastrophe. After an unprecedented shift to clean protein, the planet has remained stable. In fact, life on earth begins to get markedly better. Looking back from a hundred years into the future, historians point to the collective efforts of individuals, entrepreneurs, and communities that pushed farmed animal protein from the center of the plate to the side of it—and then off it entirely.

We paid attention to the medical science that linked meat consumption to degenerative diseases, and, with the surge in entrepreneurial efforts to create new and more widely available options for clean protein delivery, the shift in diet came. Before long, clean protein alternatives were cheaper and tasted better than traditional animal-based options. The change was as dramatic as it was swift, and with it came a precipitous drop in heart disease, cancer, diabetes, obesity, and Alzheimer's disease. We were living healthier and longer than ever before. The cost of health care plummeted, and the world economy flourished.

Governments and nonprofits seized the possibility of clean protein as not just the answer to poor health and crippled economies but as a solution for climate change. Galvanized by studies revealing that the animal agriculture industry was responsible for more greenhouse gas emissions than the transportation sector, we ended taxpayer subsidies for animal products and invested in clean protein alternatives. Rainforests regenerated, and subsistence farmers returned to their land. Aquifers were replenished, as was nature's biodiversity.

As people shifted toward healthier and more sustainable clean proteins, our natural compassion for animals asserted itself in all aspects of our lives. We saw animals as friends and coinhabitants of our planet, not as dinner. The limited number of farm animals who remained were treated well, with strong laws and international treaties to protect them from egregious abuse. A spirit of oneness graced the collective soul of humanity.

Unlike the Mesopotamians, the Mayans, and the Romans, we were able to use our collective will to survive what many were predicting would lead to yet another fall. We summoned our better angels, banded together, and collaborated in our salvation. We convinced those who thought change was too expensive, who refused to believe a dinner plate could exist without a steak, a bun without a hot dog, a Thanksgiving table without a turkey that had been raised and slaughtered for food. We proved them wrong and then we invited them to share our new, happier, more peaceful world.

And it was wonderful.

Acknowledgments

This book has taken shape because of the many people who sensed the restless and relentless spirit of change in the air, and said Yes to it. Georgina Levitt and Amanda Murray of Hachette Books; they took seriously the cultural obsession which is "protein" and let us explore and report back. We are lucky to have had Jennifer Rudolph Walsh, our agent from WME, work with us on the thesis, honing it until it was right.

A huge and hearty thank you goes out to Chef Jason Wyrick, who not only contributed many of the protein-rich recipes in this book, but who also edited the entire recipe section, all while running his food business and writing his own book; this because he passionately believes that good food can be the cure. Thank you to all the chefs, superstar personalities, and food entrepreneurs who shared their recipes and advice herein; you make Clean Protein delicious.

Thank you to Heidi Bassett Blair for not only being a believer in the future of protein, but for orchestrating the super-fun photo shoot, and for making us look way cooler than we actually are! And to Kari Castrogiovanni for lighting, editing, and tweaking the final shots.

We would like to thank our research interns for their diligent and hard work: Rebia Khan, Emily Fox-Penner, Lena Tachdjian, and Tati Freiin von Rheinbaben. We would also like to thank Dr. Michael Greger for helping to keep us on the scientific straight and narrow and Toube Benedetto for her expert editorial assistance.

Thank you to Cisca Schreefel who, with the best organizational calendar we've ever seen, skillfully steered the book to delivery. Carrie Waterson, the copyeditor whose keen eye shaped the manuscript so that it became evermore clean and clear. To our text designer, Trish Wilkinson, who made our words easy on the eyes. Gratitude goes to Richard Aquan for the cover design. Thank you to the Hachette sales team who, from the inception of this project, believed in the message of Clean Protein, and thus fanned the flames of a revolution. And gratitude to Mollie Weisenfeld for fielding all the communication and details.

Bruce would like to thank Kathy for inviting him to write this book with her; your generosity and good humor are boundless, and my debt to you is deep. Chapters 10 and 11 cover the focus of Bruce's work with The Good Food Institute (GFI), which would not have been possible without the wisdom and support of a lot of people, most importantly Nathan Runkle, Nick Cooney, and Vandhana Bala for conceiving the idea of GFI and serving on our board. To David Wolfson and the entire team at Milbank for your endless and brilliant legal support. To Josh Balk, Kathy (again), Paul Shapiro, John Mackey, David Reuben, Matt Ball, and Peter Singer for your unwavering support both for GFI and for me personally. To the stunningly impressive leadership team at Mercy For Animals for carrying the early weight of forming GFI and to the equally impressive GFI staff and advisors (see gfi.org /our-team) for making every day at "work" deeply meaningful and self-actualizing. And to our earliest and staunchest supporters, including Ryan Fletcher, David Bronner, Mike Bronner, and our

Dr. Bronner's family; Chuck Laue, Jennifer Laue, Lisa Feria, and Kathy Lowery; Ari and Becky Nessel; HRH Prince Khaled bin Alwaleed; Alinta Hawkins; Lewis Bollard and The Open Philanthropy Project; Jeremy Coller and Rosie Wardle; Leigh Bantivoglio; Suzy and Jack Welch; Loretta and Chris Stadler; Timi and John Sobrato; Kathy Head; an anonymous foundation that has offered both philanthropic support and extremely useful guidance every step of the way; and among the most generous people I have ever met, an amazing anonymous donor in the Garden State who made the whole GFI endeavor possible. Finally, I thank Alka, the love of my life and my inspiration.

Kathy thanks Bruce for being her mentor, teacher, friend, and now co-writer; I am forever awed by your ethically driven intelligence, unwavering generosity, and seemingly endless ability to get "stuff" done. And lastly, I nod to my love and life-partner, Dan Buettner; let's go sit on the porch, drink some wine, and relax for a little while.

Suggested Resources

There is a limitless number of books, websites, films, and other resources about shifting toward a more plant-focused diet. Rather than simply giving you a long list, we have narrowed our favorites down to just a few in each category that represent a very good start; if you work your way through our suggested resources and would like more, please check out our websites, KathyFreston.com and gfi.org.

HEALTH

How Not to Die: Discover the Foods Scientifically Proven to Prevent and Reverse Disease, by Michael Greger, MD.

Prevent and Reverse Heart Disease: The Revolutionary, Scientifically Proven, Nutrition-Based Cure, by Caldwell Esselstyn, MD.

Eat More, Weigh Less: Dr. Dean Ornish's Life Choice Program for Losing Weight Safely While Eating Abundantly, by Dean Ornish, MD.

The Whole Foods Diet: The Lifesaving Plan for Health and Longevity, by John Mackey, Alona Pulde, MD, and Matthew Lederman, MD.

The Pleasure Trap: Mastering the Hidden Force That Undermines Health and Happiness, by Douglas J. Lisle, PhD, and Alan Goldhamer, DC.

The China Study: The Most Comprehensive Study of Nutrition Ever Conducted and the Startling Implications for Diet, Weight Loss, and Long-Term Health, by T. Colin Campbell, PhD, and Thomas M. Campbell, MD.

NutritionFacts.org

PCRM.org

TheVeganRD.com

LIFESTYLE

Quantum Wellness: A Practical and Spiritual Guide to Health and Happiness, by Kathy Freston.

The Lean: A Revolutionary (and Simple!) 30-Day Plan for Healthy, Lasting Weight Loss, by Kathy Freston.

Lighter.World

OneGreenPlanet.com

VegNews.com

VegWorldmag.com

ForksOverKnives.com

Rich Roll podcast

COOKBOOKS AND RECIPES

The No Meat Athlete Cookbook: Whole Food, Plant-Based Recipes to Fuel Your Workouts and the Rest of Your Life, by Matt Frazier and Stepfanie Romine.

Vegan Mexico: Soul-Satisfying Regional Recipes from Tamales to Tostadas, by Jason Wyrick.

Crossroads: Extraordinary Recipes from the Restaurant That Is Reinventing Vegan Cuisine, by Tal Ronnen.

Quick-Fix Vegetarian: Healthy Home-Cooked Meals in 30 Minutes or Less, by Robin Robertson.

WickedHealthyFood.com

hotforfoodblog.com

TheFeedFeed.com

MinimalistBaker.com

OhSheGlows.com

ANIMALS

Eating Animals, by Jonathan Safran Foer.

Animal Liberation, by Peter Singer.

Dominion: The Power of Man, the Suffering of Animals, and the Call to Mercy, by Matthew Scully.

Living the Farm Sanctuary Life, by Gene Baur and Gene Stone.

Why We Love Dogs, Eat Pigs and Wear Cows, by Melanie Joy, PhD.

VIDEOS/FILMS

Forks over Knives

Cowspiracy

The Ghosts in Our Machine

What the Health

Recipe Index

General Index